How to Stop
SMOKING
Now, and Forever

howtobooks

Please send for a free copy of the latest catalogue:

How To Books
Spring Hill House, Spring Hill Road,
Begbroke, Oxford OX5 1RX, United Kingdom
info@howtobooks.co.uk
www.howtobooks.co.uk

How to Stop SMOKING
Now, and Forever

Read this book right through before making the final break – and you'll quit for good.

REVISED AND UPDATED · 2ND · SECOND EDITION ·

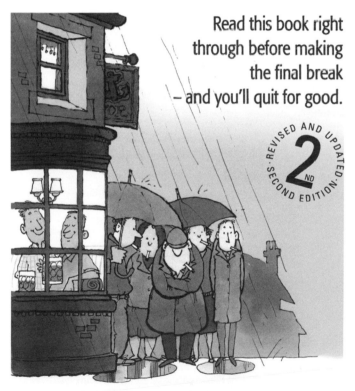

Dr HARRY ALDER and KARL MORRIS
with Dr Dev Shah

howtobooks

Published by How To Books Ltd,
Spring Hill House, Spring Hill Road,
Begbroke, Oxford OX5 1RX. United Kingdom.
Tel: (01865) 375794. Fax: (01865) 379162.
info@howtobooks.co.uk
www.howtobooks.co.uk

The right of Dr Harry Alder and Dr Karl Morris to be identified as
authors of this work has been asserted by them in accordance with the
Copyright, Designs and Patents Act 1988.

British Library Cataloguing in Publication Data
A catalogue record for this book is available from the British Library

ISBN 978 1 84528 223 3

Cover design by Baseline Arts Ltd, Oxford
Produced for How To Books by Deer Park Productions, Tavistock
Typeset by PDQ Typesetting, Newcastle-under-Lyme, Staffordshire
Printed and bound by Cromwell Press Ltd, Trowbridge, Wiltshire

NOTE: The material contained in this book is set out in good faith for
general guidance and no liability can be accepted for loss or expense
incurred as a result of relying in particular circumstances on statements
made in the book. The laws and regulations are complex and liable to
change, and readers should check the current position with the relevant
authorities before making personal arrangements.

Contents

Foreword
by
Dr Chris Hardy, Consultant Physician in Respiratory Medicine, Manchester Royal Infirmary

I work as a Consultant Physician with a speciality in respiratory medicine. On an all too regular basis I see the terrible consequences of smoking on a person's health and well-being.

I also have first hand knowledge of many, many people who desperately want to stop smoking; have been told to stop smoking by their GPs or specialists, but find that they cannot, even after trying numerous conventional methods. Millions of people want to quit, millions of pounds are spent trying to persuade them to quit; even more millions are spent treating those who don't quit for smoking-related illnesses.

As smoking is a learnt behaviour (we are not born smokers) it is quite clear to me that there is a major psychological element to quitting cigarettes as well as the more widely accepted chemical dependency issues. But very few people have the specific knowledge required to change a habit at the necessary unconscious level of behaviour.

I feel that the information contained in this book gives priceless knowledge to the smoker who genuinely wants to be rid of this terrible habit – it is in effect *the missing link* in the area of smoking cessation.

The research is sound, the techniques simple and I am sure that if the procedures recommended are followed then the results will be impressive.

This is not a quick fix, no effort, all-things-are-easy type of book. This is a genuinely effective intervention for those people who are serious about wanting to quit their smoking habit.

I am aware of the work of the two authors Dr Harry Alder, a prolific writer and expert on the mind-body connection and NLP, and Dr Karl Morris, a practising therapist and psychologist. Contributor to the book Dr Dev Shah is a registered pharmacist and has been involved in the dispensing and prescribing of smoking cessation products for many years. I recommend that you read this ground-breaking book, understand the information and then take action. You will never regret being a non-smoker.

Dr Chris Hardy
Manchester Royal Infirmary

You Can Do It

You can become a non-smoker if you want to. It doesn't take long, it doesn't hurt and it is permanent if that's what you want. This book and the desire to stop is all you need – no need for nicotine replacement therapy (NRT), drugs or other products. For the first time this book sets out the key elements of successful cessation in a systematic way.

Most attempts to stop smoking last for about 24 hours. Mark Twain said it was easy to give up – he had done it thousands of times! According to the US Department of Health and Human Services little more than 2 per cent of smokers successfully quit each year. Similarly, in the UK, the NHS Centre for Reviews and Dissemination says that 'health professional advice about quitting can achieve cessation rates of 2 per cent'. After 24 hours, about two-thirds resume smoking. If you have tried and failed, you are certainly not alone.

These estimates conceal the fact that thousands of smokers give up – without pain or trauma – successfully, and permanently. We know why and we know how, and that's what this book is about. Quite simply, with the right knowledge and know-how anyone can give up once and for all, with far less stress and physical discomfort than most smokers have experienced repeatedly in their previous, failed attempts.

Notwithstanding the dismal statistics, smokers are giving up in increasing numbers, especially in the western, most developed world. One report estimated that one half of all people who have ever smoked have now quit. Smoking-related cancer and other diseases have fallen amongst young men both in the UK and the USA. Yet at the same time many thousands of smokers try and fail, as regularly as weight watchers, and with little more success than most of us have with New Year's resolutions.

Those still hooked face increasing social isolation, if not pariah status, especially from ex-smokers. Apart from youngsters starting out – who have hardly come to terms with the idea of death and fatal diseases which they associate with older people – just about every smoker, in their heart of hearts, wants to quit. Some 80 per cent in the UK and 70 per cent in the USA *say* they do when questioned. But that doesn't tell the full story. For instance, strangely, even those who say they enjoy the 'habit' (we will use that term for the time being), when interviewed say they tried to give up at some time in the past. And, to the very last smoker, they would prefer to get their 'pleasure' without all the nasty downsides. Very few smokers nowadays are not aware of the main dangers, but research has shown that on average they underestimate the degree and range of the risks they take and this reduces their commitment to quit.

The good news for smokers is that science and common sense have provided the solution. It is all a matter of:

- the right information
- a proper understanding of all the issues involved
- and some specific know-how about making the necessary changes.

This sort of knowledge, however, has been slow to percolate down to the desperate smoker who wants to give up. This book makes it easier than you might ever have imagined and includes all the information and guidance you need. Given the great volume of information on the subject, we don't major on *why* you should give up unless it impinges on the actual process and your chances of success. We concentrate, rather, on *what to do and how to do it*.

One thing is certain: no single formula, system or product will do the job. That is why so many attempts fail. On the contrary, some important principles underlie what for most readers will mean a major life change, and you will have to make changes on several fronts to ensure a solution for life. In particular, giving up a lifetime habit will mean a change of mind – a different way of thinking. But leave that to us for the moment – that is part of our purpose in writing the book. As we introduce the subject and the approach you will take, start to look forward to all the benefits of becoming a non-smoker for no less than the rest of your life.

You have probably acquired plenty of facts over the years. The evidence of the harmful effects of smoking on health and well-being, for example, is now unequivocal. And 'harmful' is a rather euphemistic way to put something on the scale of a major war, with as many personal tragedies. Relatives and friends enduring the horrific final stages of lung cancer, emphysema and other smoking-related diseases are only too aware of the personal suffering and tragic waste of life. Smokers and non-smokers alike share these pains when it affects their family or work place. Children may suffer particularly when relatively young parents or grandparents are affected. A UK study of over 10,000 survivors of heart attacks showed that smokers in their 30s and 40s suffered five times as many heart attacks as non-smokers. At a personal as well as global level the case against smoking is well documented. But most readers will have made the decision to quit anyway – or at least desire to do so – and simply want help in actually doing it.

It seems that only the large cigarette companies, faced with record litigation, continue to attempt any self-justifying case. Less apparent though, governments around the world have come to depend on cigarette tax revenues, and most act more sluggishly in prevention and cure than their health warnings might suggest. Even with the full scientific facts at their disposal, some governments remain strangely mute amidst the acrimonious debate and the rising power of consumer movements. Most intelligent smokers realise that powerful advertising, and mixed messages from governments and the media, support the smoking status quo because of an imbalance of vested interests. But that doesn't stop any smoker from doing what they want to do once they are informed. The 'science and technology of smoking cessation' speaks for itself.

> The UK suffers thousands of deaths every year through road accidents, accidents at home and at work, murder and manslaughter, suicide, poisoning, overdoses and HIV infection. Smoking kills around six times more people than *all these put together.*

Public attitudes in western countries are increasingly polarised against the smoker. The state of California – a trendsetter in the USA, if not the world – has banned smoking in public places. This is part of a trend in which the range of public non-smoking environments, such as restaurants and shopping malls, gradually increases. Both smokers and non-smokers vote with their feet, of course, in cases such as restaurants. The trend towards a total ban, rather than a separate, ventilated, non-smoking section, for instance, seems irreversible. As the barriers get higher, in many cases backed by legislation, smokers have to invent ever more ingenious self-justification for their 'pleasure'. Social pressures don't make it easier to give up, however. They just add to the stress and low self-esteem of the embattled smoker and his or her consequent need for another fix.

Shock advertising programmes don't seem to work and are often counterproductive, especially among teenagers. Even full, technical awareness of the cancer, heart disease and other medical facts doesn't make much impact. You can still see smokers puffing away at the main entrance to hospitals and company offices. General medical practitioners themselves don't set a good example either, when it comes to smoking statistics. The exception in the medical profession, interestingly, is those who specialise in smoking-related diseases and see the consequences at closer hand. Paradoxically most smokers accept the antisocial – and even the inevitably evil – nature of smoking. Yet they remain hopelessly dependent on the habit, although in most cases not for want of trying. Thus increasingly latter-day smokers live a lie, more in the way we associate with alcoholics and addicts of hard drugs.

So we have the paradox: smokers say they enjoy it but repeatedly try to give it up. They say they want to give up but don't seem to make any serious attempt to do so. They usually have a few stock 'reasons' for their continuing behaviour, and we will address some of these in Chapter 4. Yet at the same time the average long-term smoker, including those who say they enjoy it, has made several failed attempts to give up. Sadly, each attempt undermines any 'reasons' they cite for smoking in the first place, and reconfirms what to them is an addiction they cannot handle. Increasing awareness of the true situation further compounds the stress of health, family and other pressures. And all this combines to fuel the habit. The prison walls get higher and self-esteem sinks lower.

In fact smoking gets *practically* harder as the years go by. For example, as the ranks of non-smokers swell, the remaining habitat of smokers gets ever smaller and more uncomfortable. The smoker's place is outside the office or hospital, in the garden, in the rain – in some 'special place', huddled together for mutual support. They find themselves squeezed out of nice places, whether by law or popular pressure. A sense of anger, desperation or guilt follows, and yet more stress. That means even greater dependence on the drug that seems to offer the only temporary relief.

All this adds to the wisdom of quitting – which was never in doubt. But it also adds to the smoker's difficulty – or perceived difficulty – in making the break. The embattled smoker now has even more pressure to contend with. And it is usually pressure of some sort that drives them to the next fix, so it can become a vicious circle of frustration and disappointment. We take all this into account, and expose some of the common smoking myths. In many cases smokers attempting to give up make it hard on themselves by sticking to old beliefs and entertaining certain 'facts' long since disproved. This happens unknowingly, of course – not just because a person doesn't have all the up-to-date information, but because the real power of the smoking habit lies in the subconscious mind. That is why rational decisions and so-called willpower have little effect. So we address the importance of the mind in all this, and especially what goes on unconsciously.

You will learn how to identify then change the various beliefs and attitudes that control smoking behaviour, in effect creating new mental programmes. You will understand the difference between the addictive and habitual aspects of smoking. Each involves very different factors and each requires a different solution. We are all different anyway, and smokers have remarkably different experiences when giving up, even when they follow the same basic methods. One thing is certain: you can multiply your chances of permanently quitting by the right information and know-how – not just about the dangers of smoking, but specifically about how to quit.

It is impractical for authors to offer guarantees, as we have no guarantee ourselves that readers will read the book carefully right through, let alone carry out what we suggest. However, based on the best scientific and technical information we now make available, if you are willing to follow the process with an open mind, you can guarantee success yourself.

Dr Harry Alder and Dr Karl Morris

1

Stop Smoking Technology

'Stop smoking technology' has increased rapidly in recent
years. As well as learning about the consequences of
smoking, we have learnt a lot about the practical question
of how to quit. Unfortunately, smokers' perceptions belie
the well-researched facts. Ignorance accounts for
unnecessary failed attempts, or reluctance to make a serious
attempt in the first place. We now have plenty of evidence as
to what works and what doesn't work. Comparisons have
been made between, for example, patches, gums, willpower,
acupuncture, various drugs such as Zyban and other
methods. A lot has been verified scientifically in large,
controlled studies. In areas where scientific measurement is
difficult, such as personal psychological factors, anecdotal
evidence is in certain cases overwhelming. More than
anything the 'common sense test' plays a big part in
whether a remedy will work in any individual situation –
not least in creating the self-belief and motivation to embark
on such an important lifestyle change. However, this
information takes a long time to reach the general smoking
public, and myths still abound.

IDENTIFYING CONTRIBUTORY FACTORS

By dividing smoking into four categories we can show some of the important factors involved, and make the process of giving up simpler. Smoking involves:

- What goes on inside your brain – the neurochemistry that accounts for addiction, conditioning and the programmes that run all our habitual behaviour.

- Stimulus response-type reflexes, like Pavlovian conditioning.

- Psychological factors, such as attitudes and beliefs about yourself and your habit.

- Social factors, such as peer pressure, work conditions, and support from partners and others.

To give up you need to know something about these factors, to help identify those that contribute to the problem in your specific case and to know where to direct your attention. You will meet them all in some form throughout the book (and they overlap), but in particular when they impinge on the giving up process. For instance, we need some background knowledge to explain why some remedies, contrary to popular understanding, are ineffective and why others, properly applied, just about guarantee success. So we can use these four categories as a high-level checklist. In some cases we will need information – the facts plus some background. In other cases we will need techniques, or know-how – such as to identify psychological factors and change them.

Do unto others

A 1990 USA Surgeon General's report concluded that passive inhalation of smoke by non-smokers was extremely harmful. A 1992 study by the USA Environmental Protection Agency (EPA) confirmed the report, concluding that second-hand smoke, defined as smoke inhaled by a non-smoker residing with a smoker, was a proven human carcinogen that caused 3,000 lung cancer deaths a year in non-smokers. The report also blamed second-hand smoke for up to 30,000 cases of asthma in children, 20 per cent of annual asthma attacks in children, and 15,000 hospitalisations of children each year due to respiratory problems. In 1992 the American Heart Association reported that passive smoke caused heart disease and aggravated pre-existing heart disease. Second-hand smoke kills about 40,000 people a year through heart disease, and it has been linked to cervical cancer, brain tumours, birth defects and sudden infant death syndrome (SIDS). Smokers seem extraordinarily insensitive to the known damage their behaviour causes to other people. Knowledge of this sort can help a smoker make the final commitment to stop, and also increase their chances of success.

Some information is more readily available than other information.Thankfully the link between smoking and lung cancer, known for many years, has eventually got through. But that is just the tip of an iceberg. Smoking causes about 20 harmful diseases, and the average smoker is not aware of the true nature of the different risks. Lung cancer, for example, accounts for a *minority* of deaths due to smoking. But this information, even when complete and accurate, doesn't address the *practicalities* of quitting.

Smokers are equally uninformed about how best to give up the habit. Consequently, in their attempts to stop, desperate smokers adopt techniques known to be ineffective.

RESEARCH AND REMEDIES

Nicotine replacement therapy
Nicotine replacement therapy (NRT), or continuing use of nicotine in other forms and at lower dosages, comes to mind first as a remedy. However, this has not been measured in terms of permanent (lifetime) withdrawal, and even using the typical six-month to one-year abstinence criterion it is not as effective as the advertising hype suggests. In light of the particular addictive properties of nicotine – whatever the dosage or method of intake – this should be blatantly obvious. Continued physical addiction is *guaranteed*, for instance, by feeding more of the addictive drug. That's the way addictive drugs work. Worse than that – the craving and stress tend to *increase* because of the lower, shorter-lasting relief. So giving up the drug gets ever harder.

Inhaling poison

Carbon monoxide replaces oxygen in the body. Cigarette smoke contains between 1 and 3 per cent carbon monoxide. Experiments show that smoking only one pack of cigarettes within an eight hour period results in a 7 to 15 per cent carbon monoxide saturation of the blood. This reduces the amount of available oxygen in the body and hinders muscle action and mental function. The carbon monoxide literally 'starves' the body of oxygen, which is vital to our survival. Carbon monoxide is an all too common poison used in suicides by means of car exhausts.

Meanwhile, cigarette manufacturers face a rearguard (though still profitable) action, as sales of NRT products such as **patches**, **gums** and **inhalers** increase apace. 'It's an ill wind...'. This illustrates the almost miraculous, all-pervasive impact of marketing on the sales of both cigarettes and so-called non-smoking remedies. 'Cures' involving such products are often short-lived, and thus meet the basic requirement of the commercial success of the product – repeat sales. Even in the case of NRT the most cited research adopts a six month cut-off point as a 'cure' or 'cessation'. But 'cessation' applies to cigarettes rather than nicotine, the addictive element in the cigarettes, which the product perpetuates. Extraordinarily, the smoking public accepts remedies that patently fail in the majority of cases, simply because they are 'accepted' remedies.

More recently on the market, **NRT lozenges** fall into the same general category, except that they contain a higher dose of nicotine, so as with all NRT products they perpetuate the physical addiction. As they can be more precisely linked to the ups and downs of the craving than patches, and involve *doing* something, these may help in replacing part of the habitual aspects of smoking, much like sucking mints does, but it is too early to judge.

Patches and gums generally claim approximate doubling of the chances of success (measured against the research period of perhaps six months). This is from a very low base line, however, and thus falls near to willpower on the withdrawal success ladder. Most significantly though, research into these products is almost always linked with some other interpersonal intervention, such as advice, counselling, or a helpline type resource. In fact, it is almost impossible to isolate remedies such as NRT from other variables such as:

- willpower
- motivation
- recourse to family and friends for support
- a recent event increasing the desire to quit
- circumstances such as a new car you want to keep fresh-smelling
- present stressful life circumstances
- a job that precludes smoking
- the smoker's immediate social circle
- a recent smoking-related bereavement
- the burden of the expense of buying cigarettes.

Widely used remedies such as patches and gums may
actually make the problem worse by perpetuating the
addiction at a low dosage that does not relieve the
withdrawal craving. Add to this the fact that the smoker
continues to incur significant cost, with nothing to show for
it in terms of withdrawal from nicotine dependency. Less
apparent, the heavy marketing of such products has a
similiar, unconscious, conditioning effect to the promotion
of cigarettes themselves – and you don't want to be hooked
on patches forever. At best this leaves the smoker confused.

Anti-depressant drugs

Anti-depressant drugs are known to help withdrawal.
Brupopion (Zyban is the best known trade name) is the most
common, and success rates of up to 30 per cent are claimed
both as a stand-alone remedy and also in association with
NRT plus guidance or counselling. In some cases there have
been disturbing side effects and it is a fairly expensive drug,
usually prescribed for a period of some months. The same
unaccounted variables as with NRT may apply.

Smokers often have other **motivation** to stop when they
undergo an expensive remedy such as this, and the effect of
this cannot be measured in the published results. As
motivation is cited universally as the single most important
factor in giving up, the results of drug-based therapies are
not reliable. In particular they do not address the habitual
behaviour and psychological factors involved. Few studies
measure effectiveness beyond 18 months in any case, so this
is not a measure of permanent withdrawal, with which we
are concerned in this book.

15

The published effectiveness measures of NRT and
Brupopion are:

> ... when combined with instruction on its use, counselling,
> and follow up. Drug therapy is not a panacea and requires
> some behavioural support in order to have optimal
> effectiveness.
>> (R. M. Davis, Healthcare Report Cards and Tobacco Measures.
>> Tobacco Control 1997; 6:S70-S77, cited in New Developments
>> in Smoking Cessation, Allen V. Prochazka.)

Other researchers make similar qualifications. For example,
Schneider *et al.* showed that mere dispensing of nicotine gum
actually resulted in a lower quit rate with active gum than
with placebo treatment (8% nicotine gum, 13% placebo
gum). In fairness, the product inserts for all transdermal
nicotine remedies indicate that it should be used as part of a
cessation programme. Of course most patients simply buy
and apply the patches like sticking plaster. Without any
behavioural help, we can therefore expect very low quit rates
with the nicotine patch (according to Allen V. Prochazka in
his article New Developments in Smoking Cessation, in the
order of 5 per cent).

Drugs are products just like cigarettes, of course, and
repetitive attempts to give up mean repeat sales and more
profit. The fact that these profits fund major research
programmes helps to explain why the truth about the
relative effectiveness of remedies does not reach the average
smoker.

Behavioural programmes

The obvious questions arise: what part of any success is due to the **behavioural support** and other interventions, and which of those different interventions were most effective? We don't have answers, and it is unlikely that any will emerge, as the miscellany of potential non-drug treatments cannot compete with the massive lobbies of the pharmaceutical industry from which NRT products and anti-depressant drugs are supplied.

A variety of behavioural cessation programmes is available. Lando *et al.* found that the quit rates with the American Lung Association and the American Cancer Society programmes were 16 and 22 per cent respectively, at one year. Of course not many smokers are willing to attend classes over a period, which this method involves, so relatively few benefit anyway. More importantly for our purposes, the key components to an effective behavioural programme that have been identified are:

- assessment of stages of change
- identification of barriers to quitting
- and development of cessation and relapse-prevention plans.

You can get all this and more from this book – it does not require behavioural classes, but straightforward information. Moreover, in most behavioural programmes, 'barriers to quitting' do not include the **major psychological factors** we cover, and which account for relapses, especially after more than a year (the cut off measurement period for the above claimed success rates).

Other approaches and remedies

Organic cigarettes
Organic cigarettes do not help. You may lose the lead and arsenic from fertilisers, but you still get the nitrosamines (that cause cancer in practically everything they touch) and carbon monoxide at maybe 75 times the dose that is any good for you, seven times the acceptable dose of formaldehyde, and about 130 times the acceptable dose of the carcinogen acroleine.

Low-tar cigarettes
Similar research conclusions have been reached about low-tar cigarettes, which are not substantially less hazardous than the high yield type. A study published by the American Cancer Society said that low-tar cigarettes offered less potential for cancer, and in fact were responsible for a type of cancer that reaches deeper into lung tissue.

Filters
Filters, likewise, do not remove enough tar to make cigarettes less dangerous. They are just a marketing ploy to trick you into thinking you are smoking a safer cigarette.

Acupuncture
Whilst a *New Scientist* article (see page 23) showed acupuncture as giving a 24 per cent success rate (more than twice that of nicotine gum), some recent research concluded

that it gave no better results than a placebo control group, a similar level to willpower.

Cutting down gradually
What about cutting down on cigarettes gradually? All the evidence suggests that this is far less likely to work in the long run than simply stopping altogether. The last few cigarettes are the hardest to give up and a smoker usually puffs on these harder and longer, so there is no real health gain and the craving may intensify. In most cases, even if you cut down the numbers will creep up again. There is obviously less constraint involved in smoking that extra cigarette than starting up all over again after a period of abstinence. So whatever logic might apply to gradually cutting down, psychologically you are probably on to a loser.

Willpower
Willpower ranks very low in the success stakes, and a little thought quickly confirms why if you refer to the checklist of cessation factors at the beginning of the chapter. The addictive aspect of smoking certainly does not respond to willpower. More importantly, the various psychological factors tend to operate unconsciously and on a different mental level. At the same time, we exercise our will in quite different ways. For example, you exercise your will when making a decision to quit, but you also need to exercise it repeatedly when faced with the temptation to light up, when

saying no to a social invitation that may weaken your resistance, when disposing of ash trays and so on.

- Willpower is a function of the **conscious mind**, but the mental programmes you need to change operate at the **unconscious** level.

People exercise different amounts of willpower in different circumstances, and we all face different kinds of stress. Having said this, the low success rate of willpower does not mean you don't need it, or that you don't need to come to a firm decision. It simply means that it alone is not enough. It involves just part of your brain, and a minor part in the cessation process.

Motivation

Motivation is considered by many experts to be the single most important predictor of successful cessation, but motivation also consists of many factors and, like willpower, people exercise it in different ways and for different reasons. For example, information about the health dangers of smoking can add to a person's motivation to give it up, as can information about how to actually quit, and the feasibility of being able to do it without trauma. You may get motivation by talking to a friend who has successfully quit, reading a book or a magazine article or listening to a radio chat show. It is common for the desire to quit to increase dramatically if a close friend or relative dies from a smoking-related illness.

At another level, people get motivated when they buy a new car to keep it smelling fresh, when changing a job where smoking is restricted, when sick, when in love with a non-smoking person, when becoming pregnant and so on – in other words whenever they perceive they have good reason or **motive**. It is the combination of many motivating factors including the motive to carry on smoking that determines the chances of success. This book covers a wide range of those factors, all of which affect actually giving up the habit.

Hypnosis

Some methods show better results. A number of major research studies into the effect of hypnosis on smoking cessation, for example, have shown long-term success rates of over 90 per cent claimed in a study by T. Von Dedenroth, based on 1,000 smokers using hypnotherapy, reported in the *American Journal of Clinical Hypnosis*. Based on a one-year follow up, an 88 per cent success rate was recorded by M. Kline and reported in the *International Journal of Clinical and Experimental Hypnosis*. Published research findings by Watkins, Sanders and Crasilneck and Hall for *Hypnotherapy* claim success rates of 88 per cent. Individual hypnotherapists widely claim success rates of over 90 per cent.

An article in *New Scientist* (October 1992) put hypnosis at the top of the list for effective treatment (see box on page 26). The headline ran 'Hypnosis is the most effective way of giving up smoking, according to the largest ever scientific comparison of ways of breaking the habit'. In fact this study included 'simple relaxation', so understated the effectiveness of the better, more focused hypnosis treatments at the time, and more so now.

Hyponosis or hypnotherapy, have not enjoyed the sponsorship of the NRT and pharmaceutical industry, so there are few large scale studies to draw upon. There is no tangible 'product', and hypnotherapists do not combine to operate as large corporations, so cannot fund long-term research costs. The aim of hypnotic intervention is for a permanent cure, of course, and it would take many years to get valid results anyway. In consequence of all this, the approach has not been adopted by the main health and anti-smoking agencies who issue advice.

As if this wasn't enough to keep hypnosis out of the smoking cessation stakes, there are special problems of methodology in conducting scientific studies. For example, scripts or the words used during trance have not been standardised, so the significance of this aspect of the treatment has not been captured. This explains why the success rates of over 90 per cent consistently claimed, but which clearly just apply to certain skilled practitioners, do not figure in larger studies including good, bad and indifferent practitioners. In some cases basic relaxation methods qualify as hypnotherapy. In other cases, while the main smoking-related habits are 'cured', because of insufficient preparation and depth others are not even addressed. Therefore, however successful the technique, any such untreated behaviour can – and usually does – result in a relapse.

Recorded success rates for smoking cessation

60%   Single session hypnosis using latest relaxation methods

30%   Suggestion hypnosis only or just listening to cassette
       tapes

29%   Exercise and breathing therapy

25%   Aversion therapy

24%   Acupuncture

10%   Nicotine gum

6%   Willpower alone

Success rates reported by the *New Scientist*, vol. 136, issue 1845, 31 October 1992.

COMMON QUITTING FACTORS

Other findings regarding smoking cessation are more surprising still and correct some common myths. For example, in cases where long-term smokers successfully quit permanently, some common factors emerge:

- They did not suffer more than very moderate physical withdrawal symptoms.

- They lost the psychological need to smoke almost immediately.

- They did not experience any of the difficulties that are traditionally linked by smokers to giving up such as lack of concentration.

- They described it as 'easy', 'painless', 'no big deal' or a 'non-event'.

In short, the smokers did not experience the pain and horrors often associated anecdotally with withdrawal. They discovered that the freedom from the stress of being a smoker, and the new-found independence in being a non-smoker, brought simple pleasures they had forgotten were even possible and indeed normal.

- The sense of freedom from cigarettes is probably the most overwhelming sensation.

- Almost all regretted that they had not done what little they had to do many years ago.

Sadly, a very large percentage of smokers are simply unaware of these findings, even after decades of published evidence in some cases. It seems the myths about stopping smoking originate mostly from smokers who *fail* to quit, rather than those who succeed, as smokers, like others, tend to justify their failures.

Common factors were at work in the case of hundreds of thousands who were once as hopelessly imprisoned by the habit as you may be, and successfully gave it up. These common factors offer keys to anyone making the break today so why reinvent the wheel? The subjects themselves, however, were not necessarily *aware* of just what happened in their mind to bring about the lifetime change. The mental processes in successful cessation is the vital knowledge that provides the key to quitting quickly, easily and permanently.

Characteristics of successful quitters

Those who succeed in quitting are much more likely than unsuccessful quitters to come to some important realisations about themselves.

- Successful quitters are typically highly dissatisfied with themselves for their smoking, perceive themselves as being overly dependent on cigarettes, and see themselves as more negatively affected by their habit than most smokers.

- They are more flexible and more strongly determined to quit.

- They make more efforts to minimise the obstacles to quitting.

- They are more willing to tolerate discomfort, but in fact have an easier time going though withdrawal than the unsuccessful quitters.

There is no magic in this approach to quitting. The solution does not lie in a wonder potion – or any physical product at all. In each case certain conditions and methods were knowingly or unknowingly followed. The solution, in every case, involves a large psychological element, and depends upon a person's attitude, beliefs and lifestyle – we are all different. It engages the whole mental process. Fortunately, the mental changes needed are all within your control – you just need to know the issues involved and how to go about it. You can start by adopting the characteristics of successful quitters in the box above. These are no more than common sense and within your control to apply in your own case.

MAKE IT EASY ON YOURSELF

With a bit of thought, there should be no surprise about quitting smoking being either relatively quick or easy:

- The physical effects of tobacco addiction vacate the body within two or three weeks. That's quick in comparison with a habit that is usually counted in years or decades, even if you add a couple of weeks to get properly prepared before making the break.

- The involuntary craving, or sense of 'something missing' (as it is often described) disappears in a few days – less time than it will take some readers to carefully read this book.

- The psychological or habitual aspects are no different to other habits and respond to simple changes in behaviour.

It is therefore more a matter of:

- **Sound information** about the habit and giving it up.

- **Self-knowledge** regarding your attitudes and beliefs about smoking, including why you started and continue. It may help to keep a smoking diary, in which you record the specific circumstances that trigger a light-up, what helps you to go for long periods without a cigarette and so on.

- **Techniques** that help the preparation and quitting process. You will learn some techniques in Chapter 5, Understanding Yourself.

- **Changing a few smoking-related habits and the beliefs that support them.** Chapter 6 explains how you can reprogramme your mind to behave in new, non-smoking ways.

- **Motivation, or the sincere desire to quit once and for all.** Unless triggered by a special event such as a bereavement, the desire to quit is usually a gradual, cumulative process. You acquire information, get to know yourself and realise that there are ways to give up that apply in your particular case.

We concentrate on these rather than extraneous facts and standard, product-type remedies. Motivation has proved to be the single most important factor in success, but even lack of motivation need not be a barrier. Your motivation will increase as you understand some simple facts and, most of all, start to imagine the benefits of success and their ripple effects in your life. Like everything else concerning the habit, even motivation is within your control. In the next chapter we will address the common questions that concern nicotine 'addiction' and smoking 'habits'.

2

Habits and Addiction

We have referred to the smoking **habit**, but we will now address two very different aspects of smoking dependency:

1. **Physical addiction.** According to the USA Public Health Service Clinical Practice Guideline *Treating Tobacco Use and Dependence*, nicotine is a very addictive drug. Some cigarette companies have themselves confirmed the addictive properties of nicotine.

2. The habits – invariably more than one – associated with smoking behaviour that tend to continue to operate automatically even when a person consciously desires to act otherwise. Although all addiction, and indeed behaviour, concerns the mind, we can call this second factor **psychological addiction**.

With a better understanding of these aspects of smoking, giving up becomes far less of a hurdle, so in this chapter we will address them in turn.

UNDERSTANDING NICOTINE ADDICTION

Nicotine is the fastest addictive drug we know of, and it can take just a few cigarettes to become hooked (on average perhaps four) and just one to become re-hooked after a period of abstinence – in fact a single puff is usually enough to undo days of abstinence. Its function in the tobacco plant is to act as a natural insecticide. It acts more quickly than a dose of heroin, although it does not have the powerful characteristics of heroin addiction which can result in criminality and more visible antisocial consequences. As we shall see though, the *speed* of the addictive stimulus is an important factor when it comes to withdrawal, so we need to take account of it.

Within seconds of puffing on a cigarette, nicotine is supplied to the brain and the craving ends. That results in the sense of relaxation that the smoker sometimes associates with the cigarette. It also accounts for any pleasurable or beneficial **association** between the immediate effect of the cigarette and the behaviour related to it – such as lighting up after a pleasant meal, or when receiving a stressful telephone call to regain some feeling of control. Those **positive associations**, rather than the physical addiction, account for the psychological power of the 'habit'.

The other side of the coin is that the effect wears off quickly – maybe within a quarter of an hour, and then you need another fix. That explains why most smokers average about 20 a day. Physical addiction is the minor part of the smoker's problem, however, and one that has long been the subject of myths. So we need to set the record straight.

Nicotine's relative weakness

Although the effects of nicotine are immediate, the addictive properties are weak when compared with many other addictive drugs. For example, most smokers sleep right through the night without a cigarette. Similarly, thousands undertake long-distance, non-smoking air travel. They can do without cigarettes, to which they are 'addicted', for up to maybe 20 hours ('because I have to'), yet cannot manage without food for the period. Others attend long, smoke-free meetings at work and somehow survive, or don't smoke when in hospital for days or even weeks. More and more public places are now smoke-free, yet by and large smokers continue to live fairly normal lives.

The point is that when circumstances oblige them to do so, and they mentally accept the fact, smokers can go without the drug for long periods, notwithstanding their 'addiction'. They don't need urgent medical attention or hospitalisation because they have overrun their dosage by a few hours, as might an insulin-dependent person for instance. Some even welcome smoking bans as it means they cut down on their unwanted habit. However, there is an important sense of 'addiction' that needs to be treated: the very *belief* that they are addicted is the glue that holds the smoking habit together.

Once you understand the true nature of nicotine addiction, this aspect of withdrawal is no big deal at all. It is perfectly manageable, however many cigarettes a person smokes and for however long they have been dependent. Successful

In 1527 Archbishop de las Casas of Spain wrote about tobacco addiction among Indians, and their reporting their inability to stop smoking.

In 1604 James I, King of England, wrote a denunciation of smoking due to tobacco's addictive effect of which his doctors had told him.

In 1669 the French Academy of Science (comparable to the USA Surgeon General Committee) held a national medical conference on tobacco's mental effects. The king's physician, Dr Guy Fagon, advised that experience had shown that tobacco use shortened human life.

On 26 March 1699 Dr Fagon reported that tobacco is 'a poison that is more dangerous than hemlock, deadlier than opium... Assuredly, when [people] try it for the first time, [they] feel an uneasiness that tells us that we have taken poison.' But continuing, soon 'all reasoning, all warning is in vain. He cannot shake off his enemy...tobacco alone becomes a fatal, insatiable necessity [addiction]...smoking is a permanent epilepsy.'

In 1798 the Surgeon General (Benjamin Rush, MD) under General George Washington during the Revolution, reported smoking's adverse mental effect.

Tobacco Addiction Data 1527 to 1998 downloads.members.tripod.com

quitters know this. It is the multiple trier-failers who tend to make a big issue of addiction. Many have known these facts all the time, but use addiction as a prop – another excuse for putting off finally giving up the habit.

GETTING ADDICTED

The remarkable thing is that people become addicted in the first place. Almost every smoker can recall his or her first few cigarettes, the nasty taste and unpleasant effects such as nausea and coughing. This reaction is to be expected with any poison – in the case of cigarette burning, some of the most potent poisons we know of. First you spit it out, and then you 'register' the experience in your memory so as not to make the same mistake again. It is nature's way of protecting us from harm.

Nicotine addiction is clearly nothing to do with pleasure, relaxation, confidence and such like, as we shall see more fully in Chapter 4. Most smokers start the habit because of social or other influences such as peer pressure. These are somehow strong enough to counter the unpleasantness of the drug, as well as (if we knew at the time) the knowledge of its harmful effects. Compare this with trying a new food for the first time. If you don't like it, you don't feel compelled to continue your displeasure, persevering until it somehow becomes bearable. Most teenagers are too independent and smart to act in such a crazy way. And even if you did – as with broccoli and sprouts for most youngsters – you would probably gain benefit from the food in terms of life and health.

Jean's recollection of her first puff on a cigarette was the typical one of disgust and revulsion. 'It made me terribly sick' she said, 'but I gritted my teeth and carried on, because everybody else in the group was smoking and at the time it seemed so grown up.' I asked her to imagine going into McDonald's for the first time and ordering her very first burger. 'Just imagine if it made you sick, do you think you would ever eat another burger?' 'No way' she responded, quizzically. I explained that when we experience something so disgusting, from then on we avoid it at all costs, even to the point of paranoia. Yet smoking cigarettes can make us feel sick and horrible yet we persevere until we can 'do it'. I then used the familiar computer analogy of a programme running in her mind that was actually out of date. The key, I stressed, is to realise that that programme *was* of value when she first started to smoke, because it somehow helped her to fit in and feel grown up. I asked her if this old, unconscious program was of value now. 'Of course not' was her immediate response, 'but I can see why I have had such a problem in the past in giving up.' For her, it put smoking in a whole new light. Fortunately it's never too late to quit, and once Jean (a 40 per day smoker) realised what was happening pyschologically, she soon kicked the habit.

This is not so in the case of nicotine or any other dangerous poison. So even when we can identify the causes, such as peer pressure, persuasive advertising and other conditioning, the idea of getting drawn into smoking in the first place still seems bizarre. A smoker gets hooked, not because of the pleasure but *despite* the displeasure. They don't start smoking for the cigarette, and, as we shall see, nor will they stop by focusing on the cigarette but rather on the benefits of being free from them.

When you first start to smoke the withdrawal symptoms are very slight or non-existent. It is during this period that most young smokers convince themselves that they can easily quit when they want to, but as the addiction grows it soon becomes harder to stop. All too soon, the person starts to act and think like an addict. By then the psychological aspects of the habit, which we cover later in the chapter, far outweigh the chemical addiction. Thence, true to an addictive personality, the smoker insists that they can give up when they really want to, that they get pleasure, there's 'no problem' and so on. This cumulative addictive effect, coupled with the social pressure when people start to smoke, explains why the drug has got such a foothold in the lives of millions of intelligent people.

Nicotine withdrawal

Although nicotine is an addictive, very dangerous, poisonous drug, it is relatively easy to withdraw from. Most smokers perceive that they are 'addicted', or that there is something about cigarettes that make it very hard to give them up.

Unfortunately, this may act as a reason for continuing –
'I'm just stuck'. That makes quitting harder than it ever
needs to be. For that reason it is important to understand
the true nature of nicotine addiction, and especially the part
it plays in the overall process of cessation. Either way:

- before you can address this part of the problem you must
  first accept that you are 'stuck' or 'dependent' on your
  habit.

It never pays to kid yourself, and certainly not in the case of
an addiction with life-threatening consequences.

This a relatively mild form of addiction. It in fact represents
a small part of the overall smoking habit and is usually a
minor factor in successful cessation. Withdrawal, as with
any form of drug addiction, involves simply stopping taking
the drug. In the case of nicotine, the process is almost
always painless although it usually involves different degrees
of physical and psychological discomfort from person to
person – for two or three days. The person usually becomes
nervous, agitated and irritable. Some say they feel a little
edgy, and others experience no discomfort whatsoever. Most
smokers are quite familiar with this sort of 'withdrawal'
discomfort, which they have experienced perhaps hundreds
of times. It is what they feel when they have to face a long
period without a smoke, or cannot buy a pack because the
shops are closed, or have to face a stressful situation
without the comfort of a cigarette. It can sometimes be
described as 'mild panic' such as a person with a phobia for

heights experiences, and is likewise psychological rather than physical.

That means you cannot use your addiction as an excuse for not giving up, but nor should you underestimate the ease with which you will get hooked again, even by smoking one cigarette. The best way to reduce that risk is to change the beliefs, habits and lifestyle that will make you vulnerable to relapse. We cover **reprogramming** in Chapter 6. You cannot separate the effects of nicotine withdrawal from the effects of changing the various habits associated with smoking. Both have mental as well as physical implications.

Fear of fear itself

Although there is no physical pain involved in withdrawal from nicotine, this aspect of dependence can cause unnecessary anxiety. Smokers sometimes dread withdrawal 'pangs' and imagine them to be an unbearable trauma, with images of the 'cold turkey' that heroin addicts suffer. Or they believe they are stuck with a physical addiction like a terminal illness that they are helpless to do anything about, so resign themselves to a life of slavery. As with macho men who faint at the sight of a small vaccination syringe, it is the anticipation or fear of pain rather than the event. Paradoxically, those who have made repeated attempts in the past usually admit that they relapsed because of a minor circumstance that triggered it, and that with better planning and *mental* strength they could easily have got through. Another day would have made all the difference. In most cases they simply cannot account for their relapse, not being aware of the other psychological factors at work that they were simply not prepared for, and which we especially address in this book.

- It is usually the stimulus-response effect of a certain situation, person or environment that starts you smoking again – not the nicotine craving.

It is important to be clear in your mind about both the nature of your addiction and what it means to give up. So-called **withdrawal symptoms** are not a feature of *giving up* smoking, but of the underlying cause – *smoking*. You get the craving *between* cigarettes, so in fact you suffer withdrawal symptoms continually, seven days a week, year after year. Whatever the withdrawal symptoms, they result not from abstinence, but from the addictive drug nicotine that creates the dependency. The proof is simple: the craving stops after a few days without nicotine.

Putting blame in the right place

Although nicotine addiction is ostensibly a physical condition, it is important psychologically who you 'blame', especially when feeling irritable in the days after you stop. If you place the blame on anything or anybody other than the drug, you will turn to a cigarette like an old friend at the first weak moment to gain the relief you perceive – however misguidedly – it provides. On the other hand, if you place the blame squarely on the cigarette you will not be inclined to turn to it when your defences are down. It is now rightly the villain – the enemy. Hence the need to come to the point at which you are not 'giving up' anything whatsoever of benefit or value – just the many harmful effects of smoking. This requires a whole change of attitude and beliefs about yourself and the smoking habit. Fortunately this change can happen imperceptibly and effortlessly as you read the book. Later you will do special exercises to ensure the old programme is fully replaced.

Earlier we compared nicotine addiction with physical hunger. The body gets all sorts of signals that it wants food, even before we really need it, for example when we see a tempting, colour photo of a favourite dessert in a restaurant, or on a busy morning we notice the time and realise it is almost lunchtime. True hunger pain doesn't come for a long time. Even the headaches we get when fasting are more likely due to withdrawal from coffee and junk food additives rather than lack of food. In practice most westerners overeat anyway, and dieting can actually prevent disease and extend life. The analogy with nicotine withdrawal is useful in several ways:

- Neither case involves serious physical pain.

- Both are affected by habits – we do them without thinking.

- In neither case are we robbed of our free will to act as we wish. We choose to eat and we choose to smoke.

We need food but certainly not harmful drugs to survive. Even when hunger involves pain it is a welcome survival

What does nicotine do?

Nicotine, the active and addictive ingredient of tobacco, is a mild central nervous system stimulant and a stronger cardiovascular system stimulant. It constricts blood vessels, increasing the blood pressure and stimulating the heart, and raises the blood fat levels. In its liquid form nicotine is a powerful poison – the injection of even one drop would be deadly. It is the nicotine, not the smoke, that causes people to continue to smoke cigarettes, but it is the cigarette smoke that causes many of the problems.

Cigarette smoke is a combination of lethal gases – carbon monoxide, hydrogen cyanide, and nitrogen and sulphur oxides, to name a few – and tars, and contains an estimated 4,000 chemicals. Some of these chemical agents are introduced by current tobacco manufacturing processes, such as to make the taste sweeter and more palatable to young people, and to increase the addictive properties. Although tobacco has been smoked for centuries, only recently has it moved from the naturally grown and dried process. It appears that in the last century the negative effects of smoking have increased, partially due to the added risk produced by the chemical treatment and unnatural processing of tobacco.

Dangers in modern tobacco products include pesticides used during growth and chemicals added to the tobacco to make it burn better or taste different.

Chemicals added to the leaves and papers to enhance burning are among the major causes of fire deaths, as cigarettes continue to burn after they have been put down. The forced burning also makes people smoke more of each cigarette in order to complete it. Sugar curing and rapid flue drying are also associated with increased toxicity of cigarettes. Kerosene heat drying contaminates the tobacco with another toxic hydrocarbon.

Other toxic contaminants in cigarettes include cadmium (which affects the kidneys, arteries, and blood pressure), lead, arsenic, cyanide and nickel. Dioxin, the most toxic pesticide chemical known to date, has been found in cigarettes. Acetonitrile, another pesticide, is also found in tobacco. The nitrogen gases from cigarettes generate carcinogenic nitrosamines in the body tissues. The tars in smoke contain polynuclear aromatic hydrocarbons (PAH), carcinogenic materials that bind with cellular DNA to cause damage. Radioactive materials, such as polonium, are also found in cigarette smoke. Some authorities believe that cigarettes are our greatest source of radiation. A smoker of one-and-a-half packs per day may be exposed to radiation equal to 300 chest x-rays a year. Radiation is a strong aging factor. Acetaldehyde, a chemical released during smoking, causes aging, especially of the skin, as it affects the cross-linking bonds that hold our tissues together.

Source: Elson M. Haas MD (excerpt from *Staying Healthy with Nutrition*, Celestial Arts)

warning, as it prevents us from not eating and eventually dying. In other words, food is life-enhancing rather than life-shortening, which is the case with nicotine. The longer we go without eating, the harder it gets, whereas the longer we go without smoking the easier it gets, as the beneficial life functions quickly start to replace the harmful effects of the poison.

Breaking habits

Because nicotine addiction is inextricably linked to the habits we associate with smoking behaviour – habits we also need to break – the true symptoms of withdrawal are misunderstood and usually grossly overstated. Giving up smoking is certainly a problem, but any problem becomes easier when you can break it down into smaller, achievable parts. Treated in this way, you can keep nicotine addiction in proportion. Thousands of one-time smokers look back on kicking their habit as a brief, painless non-event that was not worth the fuss.

The method for treating nicotine addiction is simple: don't smoke for three days. More importantly, don't stop until you understand the effect of smoking habits and how you treat these. *Psychological* addiction, and the habits surrounding it, is by far the most important aspect of giving up and that is what we will now address.

HANDLING HABITS

The habits associated with smoking can be many, and include any habitual behaviour or situation linked with the practice of smoking. For example:

41

- what you do with your hands
- what you do after a meal
- what you do before a staff meeting
- what you do when receiving a telephone call from a particular person
- an image, a sound
- a time of the day, such as first thing in the morning and last thing before bed
- a place, such as a pub, restaurant, car or waiting room
- any familiar, innocuous aspect of a person's life.

All sorts of stimuli like these can trigger habitual smoking behaviour. To be forewarned is to be forearmed, so start to consider these sorts of associations in your own life, and be ready to write them down.

Smoking-related habits have to be treated differently to the physical addiction we covered earlier. Each habit has to be replaced with another habit that provides the same benefits or fulfils the same function or 'intention' in a better way. This replacement habit can be any legal activity that does not reinforce the smoking habit. At one level it may mean sucking sugar-free wine gums, drinking fruit juice, twiddling a pencil or breathing deeply. At another level it may mean missing out a regular pub stopover with smoking friends, at least for a few weeks. In every case it will mean:

- **identification** of the associated habit
- and **preparation** for the period following your last puff.

That should have already started as you read with an open mind and reflect on the reasons why you might have become dependent on cigarettes.

Habits are an integral part of the way we live and we don't like a vacuum, or sudden changes. Hence the need to *replace* them with different activities – new habits that preferably bring their own pleasure and benefits as well as replacing unhelpful habits. For example, social smoking time might be replaced by time with your children, enjoying a hobby, or studying for a qualification to help your job prospects.

Smoking-related habits may be numerous and of very different types, but fortunately the methods for changing them are fairly standard as you will see in Chapter 6. So you can eliminate them one by one, which makes changing the most ingrained habit feasible. You can start with the easy ones, and gain practice as you carry on. You can then use your habit-changing skill in many other ways. For many people giving up smoking opens a doorway to many other possibilities in their life. Smoking is rarely the only habit a person can well do without, so there can be real bonuses in addition to all the benefits of giving up the smoking habit. For instance, you will benefit by an increase in confidence as you start to take control of your behaviour and live the life you want to live.

Psychological conditioning

We have seen that nicotine addiction is mainly physical and a relatively minor factor when it comes to withdrawal.

Habits, on the other hand, are mainly psychological and are absolutely critical to permanent cessation. Having said that, physical addiction has its own psychological effects, such as convincing the smoker that he or she is hooked, providing an excuse or prop for not being able to quit, or creating images of unavoidable, painful 'cold turkey'. At the same time, ordinary physical behaviour can create a self-fulfilling mental programme. If you act really depressed, for instance, you will soon feel that way. This is illustrated in the old conundrum, 'Do I whistle because I'm happy or am I happy because I whistle?' Smoking behaviour can create beliefs out of all proportion to the true nature of the physical addiction. These beliefs, plus the automatic, reflexive behaviour they support, create the long-term habits that make a person a smoker. This aspect of the problem is not a matter of chemical dependence, but psychological conditioning.

Actual behaviour has another mental effect that we do not usually consider as psychological. Habits controlled in the mind obviously involve physical behaviour – we *live out* our beliefs or mental 'programmes'. A smoker *acts out* his or her identity as a 'smoker', and beliefs such as 'it helps me relax' or 'I can't give it up'. In turn we create new mental programmes by what we actually do. If you do something repeatedly over a period, for example, you will establish a sort of 'muscle memory'. That's how we acquire all sorts of skills. In fact muscles don't have a memory – memory happens in the brain. It just means you will be able to carry out the behaviour 'without thinking'. It *becomes* a skill, or habit – however you want to describe it – whether you intended that or not. In practice, therefore, the mind and body are interdependent and part of the overall, single system. The mind-body system operates more like two sides of the same coin. In the case of an unwanted habit like smoking, this is a vicious circle. It can only be reversed by changing the whole system or programme – what you do, and what happens in your mind that controls what you do.

Both physical addiction and mental habits therefore need to be tackled from these rather different, physical and psychological standpoints. This is because of the way our mind-bodies work, in an holistic, interdependent way. This important approach may well determine whether you will do a good, permanent job in changing the habit, so it is worth getting it clear from the start.

- We can only do anything (act, or behave) according to an instruction from the brain. In other words, all behaviour is controlled or masterminded in the mind.

- Conversely, whatever we do physically has an effect on our mind. Mind and body each affect the other.

Specifically, if you keep doing the same things (smoking-related behaviour) you will run the same mental programmes that cause the psychological addiction. We saw earlier that we treat the physical addiction simply by what we do or don't do. It is now obvious that we need to treat smoking habits not just by doing or not doing things but by *thinking* differently. In other words, by running different mental programmes.

KNOWLEDGE AND KNOW-HOW

Both these aspects of dependence – physical addiction and psychological conditioning – affect the chances of successful, permanent withdrawal. Importantly, with both approaches, and contrary to the myths, withdrawal is relatively easy. You simply need to address each aspect, first separately – because they are very different conditions – and secondly, in the right way. So you need:

- **Knowledge**, for instance about what addiction means and how habits are formed, and self-knowledge concerning your attitudes and beliefs regarding smoking and giving up.

- **Know-how**, such as how to relax and communicate with your unconscious mind in order to identify old habits and replace them with new, more helpful ones.

The more appropriate your knowledge and know-how, the easier it will be to give up the smoking habit once and for all. You have heard the expression 'a little knowledge is a dangerous thing'. When it comes to giving up smoking, incomplete knowledge (including some of the myths we have met) means you are likely to fail. Worse still, you will have another failure to cope with next time.

So here is the addiction/habit position in a nutshell:

- one fast-acting but relatively mild physical addiction, plus a few habits that create psychological dependency.

You have different aspects of the 'total habit' to attend to, but each is straightforward and completely painless when you have the right information and know-how. In Chapter 6 you will learn more about mental programmes and how to change them to become a non-smoker. By then you will have learnt a lot more about yourself (Chapter 5) and what it really means to give up (Chapters 3 and 4).

For the moment, think about what sort of activities or situations trigger or stimulate your smoking behaviour.

- What immediately causes you to light up?
- What lets you know it is time to smoke?
- What situations increase the likelihood of you smoking?

Identifying these is half the problem, as you will learn powerful techniques to 'anchor' these actions to more useful behaviour.

3

Giving Up

Most smokers say they want to give up, but they don't. Many have already tried and failed. As we have seen, the symptoms of actual nicotine withdrawal are typically mild and painless, so this alone cannot account for the difficulty smokers face when giving up, and the high failure rate. We also know that the habits linked to smoking behaviour can be changed like any other habits – again without pain or trauma. It seems there is a gap in information and understanding. This blind spot particularly relates to the psychological aspect of dependency – **the role of the mind**. In this chapter we will explain some of the psychology of giving up – why it seems so hard to most people, what happens in the brain, and so on.

JUSTIFYING SMOKING

What do smokers say? 'It helps me concentrate, or relax.' 'I get pleasure.' 'I'll put on weight if I stop.' Smokers often include one or more of these in what they will 'lose', or give up, and the *fear* of that perceived loss adds to the hurdle of quitting. Even when a person has made a firm decision to quit, sometimes outdated beliefs such as these linger and unconsciously affect their behaviour. So it is better to address each of these common smoking 'justifiers' anyway, even if they don't seem to apply in your case.

Other benefits are claimed. For instance, some claim that smoking relieves boredom. But – think about it – any honest smoker could think of 101 useful, or at least harmless, things they could do to relieve boredom (ask your spouse or partner, or boss at work). So although we shall find that the above fears of loss are illusions anyway, what you learn about them will also apply to the boredom illusion and many other less common pretexts smokers use for not giving up. The ones we have quoted are representative. Most important, the methods you will learn about *changing* beliefs like these apply universally, so your particular situation will be fully catered for. In this chapter we will consider the psychological and practical aspects of giving up.

In the chapter that follows we will deal in more detail with the above common difficulties that smokers say they contend with, as these describe specific mental programmes which you need to change.

THE GIVING UP HURDLE
Strangely, smokers usually discount all the bad things they will give up along with cigarettes, such as poisons and lethal diseases. Instead they concentrate on the above kinds of losses, or sacrifices as they see them. That is not to say they are not aware of the health and other dangers. In fact, awareness of the risks of smoking generally – although underestimated – is high in western countries. Rather, the value they place on the benefits they attribute to smoking, such as relaxation and concentration, which they fear they will lose, is somehow great enough to *outweigh* all the well-

known lethal risks. Add to that the day-to-day disadvantages of being a smoker in an increasingly non-smoking world. For example, the sense of isolation, feelings of guilt, the constraints on travel and public places, ostracism, the sense of dependence and even slavery to the drug, that worrying cough, the lethargy and – adding insult to injury – the penal cost in money you could do better things with. This is what 'giving up' means. It's because of the lopsided reasoning on the part of smokers – whether due to ignorance of the facts or beliefs that operate subconsciously – that we need to concentrate first on any 'reasons' for not giving up.

These vary from smoker to smoker, of course. Answers to the question 'What am I giving up?' may have already occurred to you, but we cover this thoroughly in Chapter 5. You will need to do your own rational evaluation as part of the process of permanently quitting. This process will not only identify some key obstacles, but will also help your motivation and resolution – an essential part of the preparation for permanent cessation.

The other side of the coin

Brian had become totally fixated on all of the problems that he would encounter when he tried to give up smoking. 'Being uptight, losing my concentration, having withdrawal symptoms, needing something to do with my hands, losing my temper' – the list seemed endless. We then started to look at the other side of the coin, and Brian conceded that he would enjoy having more money in his pocket to do the things that he really wanted to do, that he would feel great as his breathing would improve and probably the chesty cough would gradually disappear. As his mind set to work, his face lit up at the prospect of being in control of something that he felt had controlled him for years – he would no longer feel like a leper at the office when he had to creep out for a crafty smoke. We then started to explore the fact that whatever you focus your attention upon expands and becomes reality. The simple truth hit him like a right hook. 'The only thing that I have been focusing on is all the things I *don't* want.' Focusing on all the supposedly painful aspects of quitting gave him no chance to get what he actually wanted. Once he started to focus on all the benefits of being a non-smoker he had turned the corner, and his new motivation towards pleasure rather than pain soon put his long-term habit where it belonged – in the past for good.

Real losses

Whatever we uncover in this process, however, there are other 'losses' that are more tangible and universal, and we can dispose of these with little controversy. For example, giving up cigarettes means 'giving up' a cocktail of nasty chemicals. The 4,000 different chemicals a cigarette generates includes, for example, 43 known carcinogenic (cancer-causing) compounds and 400 other toxins. So even if smoking did offer benefits, there is more than enough to outweigh them when making the decision to stop or carry on. The following list covers just some of the more well known poisons:

- ammonia: household cleaner
- angelica root extract: known to cause cancer in animals
- arsenic: used in rat poisons
- benzene: used in making dyes and synthetic rubber; linked to leukaemia
- butane: gas, used in lighter fluid
- carbon monoxide: poisonous gas as in car exhausts, and a popular suicide method
- cadmium: used in batteries; linked to lung and prostate cancer
- cyanide: well known deadly poison
- DDT: a banned insecticide
- ethyl furoate: causes liver damage in animals
- formaldehyde: used to preserve dead specimens and embalming
- hydrogen cyanide: used in gas chambers
- lead: poisonous in high doses, and outlawed as a constituent in many products
- methoprene: an insecticide
- methyl isocyanate: its accidental release killed 2,000 people in Bhopal, India in 1984
- naphthalene: ingredient in mothballs
- nickel: causes increased susceptibility to lung infections
- polonium: cancer-causing radioactive element.

These – just for starters – are some of the real losses when you give up smoking.

The words 'giving up' offer a clue to why smokers repeatedly fail to change their behaviour.

- As long as a smoker thinks that he or she will have to give something up *of value*, the chances of quitting are considerably reduced.

- They view giving up as a sacrifice and a personal cost. And that smacks of willpower – a function of the conscious mind – which happens to be one of the least effective methods of quitting.

A sense of giving something up is a major psychological hurdle and applies at different mental levels:

Logical
For example, in some cases a person will offer what they consider to be logical arguments and examples about how smoking helps them to concentrate, feel relaxed and so on. They need to convince *themselves* to explain their behaviour.

Anecdotal
Sometimes they rely on anecdote, such as Aunty Mary who smoked until she was 95 and died peacefully in her bed, or 'anybody can be run over by a bus'. Strangely, in other aspects of their lives they know quite well that individual cases do not affect the true probability of events.

They will usually argue that what seems like black is white, to an ex-smoker or non-smoker, to justify their continued behaviour. And they will resent any suggestion that they are deluded, brainwashed or acting irrationally. This is a common feature of any form of addiction, such as alcohol, heroin or gambling. A lot of self-deceit is involved, and smokers themselves admit this – but usually only after they have kicked the habit. This does not imply any moral judgement. It simply illustrates the way our minds work in many situations, especially at an unconscious level, not unique to smokers. The logic of the conscious mind will always try to 'explain' the illogical behaviour rooted in the unconscious mind.

The mental control room

This psychological blind spot usually confirms a subconscious desire to continue smoking, for whatever reason. It is at this subconscious level of the mind that apparently irrational habits and psychological dependency occur. The mental 'control room' that governs our habitual behaviour lies in the deep subconscious mind rather than in the rational, logical, conscious mind. The large majority of all our behaviour falls into this 'below the surface' category. We do it automatically, without thinking. Indeed, we depend on this kind of habitual behaviour – whether boiling a kettle or getting dressed in the morning – to survive and live a normal life. It's only when what we *actually do* is contrary to what we consciously *wish to do* that conflict arises.

The answer is to change your behaviour, change your wishes, or both. Otherwise, your conscious mind will make the best *excuses* for what it knows is a fact. On the foundation of such excuses a smoker slavishly continues to smoke, contrary to all the outside evidence against the habit, and even against their own better judgement.

Typically, they maintain that it gives pleasure, helps concentration and so on. The more irrational the behaviour seems to be (as knowledge of the dangers increases, for instance), the more ingenious will be the 'reason'.

Most smokers are afraid to quit. This fear does not operate at a conscious, rational level, but fear rarely does. It is a more primeval aspect of our minds. Amazingly, the fear usually at work when giving up is not fear of sickness, disease, death, bereavement or life-threatening situations. Most smokers know the lethal dangers of smoking, but somehow all that doesn't register as fear, and it rarely stops them indulging their addiction. Rather than fear of some future mortal pay-day, it's a fear of losing – giving up – something they *have*, although they are not sure what. It is fear of losing something immediately – the moment they stop – rather than of something in the distant future like emphysema and cancer, or a few years at the end of your life. It is another function of the unconscious mind – you don't need to 'try' to be afraid, or even consciously realise that you are. This fear of some unknown loss is the response to the unconscious programme running always in the background that says 'smoking is of value'. The reality is that 'giving up' doesn't involve giving up anything of true value at all. Ironically, the belief that you are genuinely sacrificing something is one of the biggest psychological barriers to 'giving up'.

What am I giving up?

Diseases and medical conditions associated with smoking: Atherosclerosis, hypertension, heart disease, coronary artery disease, peripheral vascular disease, myocardial infarction, stroke, polycythemia, increased infant mortality, low birth weight in infants, Alzheimer's disease, vitamin/mineral deficiencies, acute and chronic bronchitis, emphysema, non-insulin dependent diabetes. Cancers: lung, mouth, skin, tongue, larynx, oesophagus, bladder, kidney, stomach, pancreas, cervix.
Allergies: rhinitis, sinusitis, various infections, burns, peptic ulcers, varicose veins, hiatal hernia, osteoporosis, periodontal disease, senility, impotence, adult acute leukaemia, adult chronic leukaemia, pneumonia, wrinkles and facial ageing symptoms, psoriasis and other skin conditions, slow wound healing.

SPLIT-BRAIN EXPERIMENTS

Fortunately this common addiction paradox of kidding oneself has been well researched and we can understand some of the strange behaviour that occurs, not just in the case of smokers, but in many situations which non-smokers will easily relate to. In particular, we have different parts to our personality – 'One part of me wants to do so-and-so and the other part finds it repulsive.' Even physiologically, we have two distinct sides to our brain – left and right – and these work in very different ways.

Roger Sperry, a joint Nobel prize winner, carried out so-called
split-brain experiments in the 1960s. Part of his work involved
dividing the right and left hemispheres of the cortex, or upper
brain. This meant cutting the *corpus callosum* – a bundle of
millions of connecting fibres – that joins them. (The patients
already suffered from severe brain seizures so had little to lose
as volunteers, and a lot to gain if the seizures could be
contained within one side of the brain.) It transpired
afterwards that the split-brain patients, whilst in most respects
normal, acted sometimes as if they now had two distinct
personalities. Without communication between the brain
hemispheres, they functioned as if with separate minds.

Sperry already knew that each side of the brain is associated
with certain main functions, or ways of operating. For
instance, the left side is involved in language, logic and step-
by-step reasoning – the sort of thinking we do consciously.
The right side is associated with spatial awareness, artistic
and musical appreciation, emotion and suchlike. The right
side, along with the so-called mid-brain, is also related to
the unconscious mind, and trance states such as when
daydreaming. It is where the smoking programmes we have
already associated with the unconscious mind happen, so we
can get some useful clues about the habit. For example, not
understanding language, the right brain is in effect mute,
and cannot communicate, either with the left brain or
through the 'articulate' left brain to the outside world. Not
surprisingly, it is often 'misunderstood' and generally has a
bad press. So, although this submerged part of the brain has
an enormous effect on all our moment-by-moment

behaviour – including smoking – it cannot always account for it or express itself.

Sperry had an opportunity to test some of these lateral brain characteristics for the first time, with what were in effect two separate brains in the same person. His remarkable experiments explain how independently our two minds can work. For our purposes it gives some insight into how smokers seem to rationalise their habit. Bear in mind that each brain hemisphere controls physical movement in the opposite side of the body. The left brain handles functions on the right side of the body (including the right hand and right eye) and, conversely, the right brain controls movement in the left side (hence the opposite side paralysis after a stroke affecting one side of the brain).

The subjects were shown images on the separate sides of the brain (via the opposite eyes), and later asked to point to another image that was related to what they had seen. One subject's left-brain was shown an image of a chicken claw, and his right brain was shown an image of a snow-covered house. When he was shown the further selection of images, he pointed to pictures of a chicken and a snow shovel. The chicken seemed fine, and on the face of it so did the snow shovel. However his *explanation* for choosing the snow shovel was that 'You need a snow shovel to clean out the chicken shed.' This was not, of course, why he chose the snow shovel, which was obviously related to the snow-covered house. But his right brain was unable to communicate the image of the snow-covered house to his verbal left-brain. It knew *without knowing why it knew* – something like intuition, another right-brain phenomenon. The left-brain, having observed the *choice*, then *made up* a reason! It concocted its own interpretation or 'excuse' for the action, but the subject did not know that he had contrived a relationship – to him the explanation seemed quite logical.

The importance of the whole mind

This kind of extraordinary response, repeated in the experiments in other fascinating ways, transformed our understanding of the way we create beliefs and habitual behaviour. As humans it is as though we cannot bear to live with *not understanding*. Everything has to have a purpose – a reason. If it hasn't, we give it one. Every smoker has their reason for smoking. Often (just like the chicken relationship) it can seem absolutely logical, although not so logical to the objective outsider. However, it is based on ignorance – or the wrong foundation. And whilst often a harmless by-product of our mental pigeon-holing, where the behaviour is harmful, such as with smoking, the 'system' can badly backfire.

The split-brain experiments illustrate the importance of the **whole mind** in making the sort of long-term changes a smoker has to make. You need to make a conscious, rational decision, but – equally important – you need to harness your unconscious mind to work in the same direction and run the new habits upon which your success will depend.

≥ENS WHEN YOU STOP SMOKING

ɛssure and pulse rate return to normal.
ɪon improves in hands and feet, making them
ᴡ...

8 hours
- Oxygen levels in the blood return to normal.
- Chances of a heart attack start to fall.

24 hours
- Carbon monoxide is eliminated from the body.
- The lungs start to clear out mucus and other debris.

48 hours
- Nicotine is no longer detectable in the body.
- The ability to taste and smell is improved.
- Nerve endings start regrowing.

72 hours
- Breathing becomes easier as the bronchial tubes relax.
- Energy levels increase.

2–12 weeks
- Circulation improves throughout the body, making walking easier.

3–9 months
- Breathing problems such as coughing, sinus congestion, shortness of breath and wheezing improve.
- Overall, lung function is increased by 5–10 per cent.

1 year
- Excess risk of coronary heart disease is half that of a smoker.

5 years

- Lung cancer death rate for average smoker (one pack a day) decreases by almost half.
- Stroke risk is reduced to that of a non-smoker 5–15 years after quitting.
- Risk of cancer of the mouth, throat and oesophagus is half that of a smoker's.

10 years

- Lung cancer death rate similar to that of non-smokers.
- Precancerous cells are replaced.
- Risk of cancer of the mouth, throat, oesophagus, bladder, kidney and pancrease decreases.

15 years

- Risk of coronary heart disease is that of a non-smoker.

Source: QUIT®

SUBCONSCIOUS DESIRES

We have referred repeatedly to the role of the subconscious mind. Although we have 'joined-up' brains, there is still a vast portion of our brain that lies outside our immediate consciousness, rather like the submerged part of an iceberg, yet which nevertheless affects most of our 'automatic' behaviour. This approximately equates to the 'mute' right brain we have just considered. It means:

- we have subconscious desires or 'intentions' that conflict with what we *consciously* desire.

For all the power of the unconscious mind, it acts in a literal, uncritical or naive way. For example, it will continue to espouse the original reason for starting to smoke – say peer pressure, living up to a social or hero image, following the crowds, etc – long after a person is ready intellectually to abandon the practice. Because we *repeated* the practice when setting out to smoke, and it seemed to fulfil our desires at the time, this part of the brain unquestioningly accepted the behaviour as being in our best interest. Unfortunately, nobody told that part of our brain that we had grown up in the meantime and got wise to the practice of smoking. Even if we consciously changed our mind, and made a definite 'decision', we did not engage the part of the brain that made the critical difference. The unconscious mind acts like a loyal slave rather than a wise adviser. This helps to explain why reason and willpower don't have much effect on a long-term smoking habit. That part of the brain simply isn't rational.

Outside conditioning

Our early internal conditioning is based on personal experience, circumstances and the vagaries of the moment, but more purposeful *outside* forces were invariably at work also. For example, the young smoker espouses the subconscious message of clever advertising that created the association of smoking with top sports people, relaxation, confidence, independence or whatever. That clinches it. The right and mid-brain absorb such messages in an unquestioning, childlike way. We thus unknowingly act out those deep beliefs that run so contrary to our better judgement – and continue to do so until we understand what is happening and know how to intervene.

In other cases outside conditioning may be more passive.

Just seeing thousands of adults smoking creates the illusion that they *must* be enjoying it. It is the lemming, or 'safety in numbers' myth – it must be all right if so many people are doing it. Many such messages are transmitted from the ambient culture to make us what we are and we absorb them like a sponge. Children whose parents smoke, for example, understandably assume that not to do so is different or abnormal. Ask yourself, how many smokers start in their thirties or forties? Usually we throw off this cultural baggage as rebellious teenagers, but in the case of smoking the conditioning continues, not so much from parents but from our peers and the big world outside. Few involve such a physically and psychologically addictive drug. Few activities have multi-million dollar advertising support and figure so prominently in cinema and the mass media.

This, in simplified form, is the psychological conditioning that makes smoking so difficult to stop. It is not the physical nicotine addiction. Nor is it the outward habits themselves, or external behaviour, which is simply the *consequence* of our beliefs and inner motivations. Hence it is not just a more complex withdrawal scenario, requiring knowledge and know-how as we have already seen, but one which takes as long as it needs to take for offending habits to be replaced.

Changing habits and beliefs

Physical withdrawal from nicotine is essentially a three-day non-event. Habits take nearer three weeks to change, and there may be several to tackle. But this is no big deal. We create new habits and give up old ones effortlessly all the time. They don't enslave us for life. This long-established 'smoker' belief system underlies our very values, identity, attitude and behaviour. In this case beliefs take the form of 'smoking helps me relax (or concentrate, relieves stress, gives pleasure)' and so on. Beliefs such as these lie at the root of the giving up problem, which is why we give them special attention in the next chapter.

On the face of it this is an insurmountable psychological problem that enslaves millions of smokers around the world. It is essential for the smoker to understand it, and it is true to say that anything 'psychological' is sure to be complex. But it is wrong to overstate it. Indeed, with the right information and know-how, and when you treat it in logical stages, the solution is simple and easy to implement:

- identify and acknowledge these beliefs
- replace them with new, harmless ones.

In this chapter we have already identified some of the beliefs that surround giving up, one or more of which apply to the vast majority of smokers. In the next chapter we will look at these in more detail. There may be others in your particular case. Some may occur to you as you read – write them down as we will refer to them later. In the light of what you now know you can address them honestly, and see them for what they are.

In short, stop kidding yourself that you have to give up anything of real value when compared with the lifetime's freedom and other benefits you will gain. This is a vital stage in the process of quitting for life, so it is worth getting it right.

$$\left(\, 4 \,\right)$$

Popular Pretexts

In this chapter we will address some of the popular reasons smokers give for not giving up:

- it helps me concentrate
- it helps me relax
- I get pleasure
- I'll put on weight if I stop.

You may have used one or more of these yourself from time to time – thousands of smokers did, who have long since given up. They didn't need brain surgery, or special psychiatric counselling, and nor do you. If they don't apply to you, read on anyway, as the psychological principles you meet will help as you identify the specific 'reasons' that apply in your particular case. Remember that we are not consciously aware of what drives most of us to smoke anyway, although this self-understanding soon emerges as we relax and 'go inside'.

THE CONCENTRATION CON
'It helps me concentrate' is a common response to the question 'Why do you continue to smoke?' Smoking itself –

cigarettes, or the nicotine in them – doesn't help concentration in any neurophysiological sense, so we need to consider the *perception* of smokers, which is what matters. Withdrawal symptoms, which start not long after finishing a cigarette, create a sense of restlessness, distraction and irritability. After a period, and especially after the shops have closed and you don't have a supply of cigarettes, or are stuck in a non-smoking environment, emotions closer to panic may set in. These are the very feelings that make it hard for the smoker to concentrate. But the fact is, it started with a *cigarette*, and got worse with each subsequent cigarette, as a vicious circle of behaviour took control. The difficulty to concentrate is *sustained* by cigarettes. In other words:

- smoking makes concentration much harder, not easier.

Why, then, the extraordinary misunderstanding? When the smoker has the next fix, the empty feeling is *partially relieved*, and for a while he or she can concentrate relatively more normally. So although cigarettes caused the lack of concentration in the first place, remarkably, the cigarette that temporarily relieved the symptoms – subconsciously at least – gets the credit. The smoker wrongly associates relief from not being able to concentrate with the cigarette because of the *timing*, and mental associations.

In fact, smoking another cigarette will never fully regain the normal brain and body function we knew as a non-smoker. Worse, it makes concentration progressively harder as the mirage of relief produces diminishing returns. Like other drugs, you need more of it to produce the same effect. Put another way – and this is the test when deciding whether to be a smoker or a non-smoker – even with the fix, a smoker will not be able to concentrate as well as a non-smoker, other things being equal, or as they did themselves before they got hooked.

- The more a person continues smoking, both in time and quantity of cigarettes, the less relief each cigarette will give. That comes with chemical addiction.

- And the less chance they have of regaining the normal level of concentration that non-smokers enjoy without giving it thought.

Even in simple physiological terms, the concentration con will not stand up. Clogged arteries resulting from smoking starve the brain of oxygen and reduce our ability to concentrate along with any other cerebral activity. Carbon monoxide, for example, which usurps oxygen, is not known as a concentration gas, simply a poison. However, the myth is powerful enough to provide a false 'reason' for continuing with the smoking habit in the face of all the evidence of the harm it causes. Fear of losing this fictitious ability to concentrate stops many people from successfully stopping. They will argue, for instance, that they need to concentrate in their job, it might affect their career, and so on.

Exposing the con
This is a self-fulfilling belief, like many beliefs. If you believe

you will lose powers of concentration without a cigarette to help, you probably will. In reality you need a clear head to concentrate, and, not least, the oxygen supply on which your brain depends. What you *don't* want, and what smoking supplies consistently, are mixed up, irrational beliefs or the nagging physical and mental craving for the very poisonous drug that caused the problem.

The concentration con is an example of the psychological addiction that makes a cigarette slave of so many people. If you still have your doubts, start to focus on why you lose concentration in the first place – why you need a cigarette, or any external prop, for your brain to function normally. If it turns out that the cigarette is both cause and cure at the same time, you need to re-examine your reasoning.

Beliefs such as this one may well operate unconsciously, of course. In other words, we would not normally express such a belief, but the *association* exists somewhere in our mind. In this case, once suspected, we have all the more reason to prise them out by introspection or include them on a list. Once we identify them they are no longer unconscious, and can be subjected to cold reason and simple common sense. Once exposed – like the visible part of an iceberg – they will no longer unknowingly hijack your decisions, and you will regain control of your life.

THE RELAXATION RUSE

The concentration excuse may not apply to you, but most smokers say that it helps them to relax. This illusion works in just the same way. The last description most people would apply to smokers is relaxed – however many they smoke a day. They can never be as relaxed as they once could be without the drug, or as relaxed as non-smokers, all other things being equal. For example, when people are relaxing after a good restaurant meal it is the smokers who are on edge. The good food, pleasant surroundings and stimulating company are not enough. They need a fix to create even a semblance of the relaxed state their friends take for granted – even between courses, as though the food part of the evening was an inconvenience. Because those relatively pleasant moments are associated in the memory with the after dinner cigarette, the cigarette gets the credit rather than the blame. Remarkably, the fact that non-smoking friends may be badly affected by cigarette smoke, and the spoiling of their pleasure in eating, does not diminish the smoker's desire to 'relax' in the only way they know how.

In the case of relaxation the physiological realities are even starker than in the case of concentration.

- Nicotine is a **stimulant** (except in certain conditions at high dosage), not a depressant.

- It speeds up rather than slows down the metabolic rate.

So relaxation is another remarkable example of the sort of irrational excuses Sperry found in his split-brain patients who tried to justify whatever in their own behaviour they could not rationally account for. In the case of smokers, the linking *corpus callosum* between the dual brains is perfectly intact. However, they have not come to terms with how the subconscious mind controls the behaviour that is set to kill them, and which they know all too well in more lucid moments is foolish, irrational and inexcusable. This frank self-awareness – a vital part of the giving up process – is sometimes referred to as **intra-personal intelligence** (intra = within). It means understanding what is going on inside, and that includes getting in touch with your unconscious mind and the hidden motivations that produce unwanted behaviour. The smoker 'relaxes' through *expectation* – conditioning and association with relaxing situations of which the cigarette happens to be a part, but, more obviously, through the deep breathing that accompanies smoking. Any sportsperson will know the effect of slow, deep breathing before an event to get relaxed – but the best effect is with fresh air rather than toxic chemicals! Nicotine, a *stimulant, reduces* the relaxing effect of deep breathing, while getting the credit from uninformed smokers.

Stress

Stress is on the other side of the relaxation coin and many smokers claim that smoking helps to relieve stress. This is another facet of the same problem. In one study, for 30 per cent of women, giving up meant more stress. One lady said that without her cigarettes she would beat the kids. In fact the physical withdrawal symptoms of nicotine are very similar to those associated with ordinary stress, which we all experience from time to time to some degree. It is this 'stress' that the smoker assumes the cigarette is relieving – 'it calms my nerves'.

A major life change

Lesley ran her own business and had a very hectic and stressful lifestyle. Her 40 cigarettes a day were 'essential' to allow her to relax and feel calm, and the very thought of being without her 'lifeline' filled her with dread and huge anxiety. Previously any attempt to quit had coincided with a personality change that made her a 'living nightmare' to work for – one of her staff had actually pleaded with her not to attempt to quit again.

We talked about how in our formative years we are conditioned to believe certain things, and about the influence of the media and advertising in particular. We discussed the fact that in the old films the stars always smoked and how they always looked so romantic, relaxed and totally in control. We discussed how to a young mind these images were hugely powerful and would provide an influence for years to come because they were embedded deep into the unconscious mind. The link to the mind became very simple: cigarettes = relaxed and in control.

I then explained that nicotine is, in fact, a stimulant, so if you are feeling stressed and uptight it should make things worse, yet the power of these long-forgotten images created the mental expectancy that smoking would make her relaxed. The expectancy is so powerful that it can even override the chemical properties in the cigarette. The look that spread over Lesley's face when she confronted the fact that she had been brainwashed all these years into believing that smoking was actually of value was truly something to behold.

In the letters I have received since the day she stopped smoking she says she can now actively question so many long-standing limiting beliefs that were imposed upon her from outside influences. So much so that she feels strongly that quitting smoking was actually a catalyst to a major life change. It brought her to totally re-evaluate her own worth and her place in the male-dominated business in which she is involved.

The simple fact is that smoking *causes* stress, not just from the continual, unsatisfied craving, but also in the various psychological pressures the smoker goes through, including guilt, low self esteem, a sense of helplessness and so on. Such inner conflict does not come without stress symptoms, and especially 'living a lie' which any addict in due course succumbs to. At best, the next cigarette suppresses the very stress that earlier cigarettes caused. Of course, deep breathing is a well known way to relax and a stress antidote, and that may partially account for the sensation (although cigarette smoke cannot compete with clean air). But even the perception of relief is only *partial* and *temporary*.

However, this is the only way the smoker knows to relax, so it is the default programme the brain always turns on when stressed.

This topsy-turvy thinking is psychological conditioning at its worst. Bear in mind that in some cases smokers have given up life partners and close friends rather than give up their addiction. The fact that they are enslaved to psychological self-conditioning rather than an incurable chemical addiction just adds pathos.

THE PLEASURE PARADOX

'I enjoy them' is a common smoker's response – sometimes the only response after the facts have been discussed. We have already explained the association between smoking and certain pleasurable situations such as a restaurant meal, relaxing with friends and so on. Relaxation, in particular, is a universally pleasurable state. It is easy to see how, once having fallen into the relaxation belief trap, smoking is then associated with actual pleasure.

The pleasure, it turns out, concerns the experiences associated with various smoking-related habits, rather than smoking itself. And the pleasure, it seems, is not a positive pleasure gained, but *the temporary avoidance of displeasure*. In fact, it is partial relief from displeasure in the form of the aggravation of withdrawal symptoms. That displeasure may be a feeling of stress, helplessness, loneliness, boredom, craving, irritation or just a sort of emptiness that has to be filled. As with the earlier associations with concentration and relaxation, the 'pleasure' comes from reverting, for a short while, to the *normal* situation of a non-smoker. It represents a hankering back to the feeling of peace and confidence that was once a normal part of life, and that didn't require drugs – the sort of pleasure you get when you stop banging your head against a wall. This is the pleasure myth:

- any 'pleasure' is only relative to the displeasure already created by cigarette dependency.

A matter of taste

The truth is that, although we once took certain pleasures to be normal, we *forfeited* them as a result of the smoking habit. Another dose of the drug partially *reduces* the loss effect, but only partially. For example, a smoker loses basic sensations such as taste due to a build up of tar and other chemicals, so much of the pleasure of a meal is lost anyway, and any number of cigarettes will not replace it. Because this happens gradually most smokers are not aware of it, just as we don't notice a gradual loss of eyesight after 40, until we get fitted with the right glasses and marvel at what we have been missing. The smoker unconsciously associates the pleasure of the good company and conversation after a meal with the cigarette, simply because the two are timed closely and fall into one mental pigeonhole.

In reality there is no way that we need cigarettes to enjoy friendship, let alone a good meal. But the fact remains that a smoker cannot enjoy such simple pleasures without a cigarette. They feel edgy, incomplete or however they describe it. So to ameliorate the harmful, antisocial effect of the cigarette, they have to smoke another one. Not only does that not solve the problem (there is still the lack of taste, still the social stigma, still the cost and still the harmful health effects) but it *extends and increases* it. It gets progressively more difficult to engage in the simplest of normal activities – like enjoying a good meal with friends – without a fix. Then, in an upside down form of logic, much like we hear from alcoholics and hard drug users who deny reality in deference to their addiction, the cigarette gets the credit for the so-called pleasure.

Ask yourself:

- What exactly is pleasurable about the cigarette?

- Is it the taste? How does the taste compare with a good meal, for instance, and why not get more pleasure from food if taste is important for 'pleasure'?

- Is it the feel of the cigarette? Ask yourself 'Are there no other feelings that give me pleasure without the many harmful effects of this drug?'

One of the biggest pluses of giving up smoking is to regain the simple pleasures you have long forgotten, and which the non-smoker takes for granted, as you once did. Cigarettes don't give pleasure. They rob you of basic pleasures.

Smoking another one perpetuates the problem, and renders simple, true pleasures even more distant and unobtainable. In one sense you will not be convinced of the pleasure you have forgone until you become a non-smoker and your senses are restored to normal, until you see the world in a truer sensory light. Then you can hardly believe how you deceived yourself – especially in crediting the cigarette with the very pleasures of which it robbed you.

Beautiful people

The association of pleasure comes in other ways. Cigarettes have figured prominently in movies featuring famous, beautiful people who seem to be living a life of pleasure and complete satisfaction. This pleasure seems to come when two people both light up, often at a romantic moment. The same sort of connotations apply to cigarette advertising, which associates smoking with something pleasurable – romance, freedom and wide open spaces, tranquillity and so on. However unsupportable – and indeed ludicrous – it packs enough psychological punch to prevent many thousands from giving up. This is mental conditioning and applies in all sorts of other areas besides smoking. The pleasure myth is a far bigger hurdle than the physical symptoms of nicotine withdrawal, and one that will take thousands of intelligent people to their grave far too soon.

We need not delve into a person's psychology to refute the pleasure illusion. Almost all smokers admit openly that they regret starting and want to give up the habit. Almost without exception, smokers do not want their children or grandchildren to touch a cigarette. Remarkably, most smokers agree with policies that restrict smoking in public places. Even the most deluded addict cannot deny the concoction of foul-tasting poisons that every cigarette contains (see page 50). They likewise admit to finding the taste awful at first, and having to persevere in *displeasure* before they could smoke regularly as the grown up people did. The destructive role of the habit is as clear as day, yet smokers continue to associate smoking with pleasure.

True pleasure

We seek pleasure in many different forms, but rarely do we seek to forgo the same pleasure at the same time – the nearest example is bulimia, in which people gorge themselves, then throw up. But this is a sad analogy for the smoker. If pushed, we can even accept that a person can enjoy something that has a foul taste, as tastes are so subjective (and people so strange), but logic breaks down when in the next breath we assert that we wish we had never indulged in the 'pleasure' and want to give it up, as is the case with smokers. Or that we want our children to be happy, but do not want them to experience the 'pleasure' we attribute to cigarettes. Or would deny the public their pleasure by restricting smoking in public places! Thankfully, most of the pleasure lost through smoking dependency, such as the taste of food, can be regained in a few days simply by not smoking. More pleasures will be regained in a couple of weeks as habits and associations gradually change and your identity as a non-smoker takes the smoker's place. Pretending that you have to sacrifice true pleasure will only delay the moment of truth and may scupper your attempt to finally quit.

THE WEIGHT WORRY

Weight gain is usually to do with the change in tastes, habits and lifestyle when you give up smoking, rather than nicotine withdrawal. People who repeatedly diet know only too well that they overeat out of habit rather than because of real hunger. In some cases it happens when a person is bored, anxious, engrossed in a problem, at home rather than at work, or when in company and so on. When withdrawing from cigarettes, there may be a tendency to nibble and eat for the sake of eating, or just to distract attention from the nicotine craving. Smokers and non-smokers alike who need to diet have to get to grips with their habits and lifestyle. We said in earlier chapters that smoking-related habits have to be replaced, not just eliminated. For example:

- If smoking gave you something to do with your hands, you will need a habit (or two) that gives you something to do with your hands, or somehow occupies your mind in an equivalent way.

- If you smoke when you are anxious, you need a behaviour that helps to reduce anxiety, such as slow breathing, relaxation exercises, visualisation or an absorbing pastime.

- If you are a reader, you will probably find you can lose yourself in an absorbing book, and this can fill up the important hours during the critical withdrawal period.

There are lots of effective methods. The trick, however, is not just to identify a wholesome replacement behaviour, but to repeat it sufficiently to form a new habit. That way you don't have to think about it or apply willpower (which at that weak moment you may not be able to muster) when the critical moment comes. It may then be too late, so the old behaviour wins out. Bear in mind that you can create *any* habit by simple repetition for a long enough period – on average about three weeks.

Good taste

Weight gain may involve another important factor. As we saw earlier, the sense of taste is one of the many functional losses associated with smoking. That means that when the addiction wears off, the taste buds start to function again, smell returns, and suddenly you are in a new world of pleasure in which even the simplest food is irresistible. To know this is to pre-empt the weight 'problem'. Otherwise, the tendency is to make up for lost pleasure and overeat. In fact the ex-smoker is in no worse a position than someone who just loves their food, and the same principles we have met apply to replacing any unwanted habits. So if weight is a particular issue – whether real or imagined – it will pay you to think about your diet in parallel with giving up smoking. Having said that, the average weight gain is just a few pounds, and most people would have to double their weight to incur the overall health risks that come with smoking!

In this case knowledge of what is happening is usually
enough, and you don't need to put on weight anyway. Once
you are aware of the tendency to enjoy food more and eat
more you can do something about it. For instance, create
whatever new habits you need to. That may mean avoiding
eating between regular meals (as millions of other dieters
do), reserving special meals as rewards for keeping to your
commitment, or for achieving work or personal goals. Or it
may simply mean eating better foods that don't pile on the
weight. You don't need to eat less in order to maintain or
lose weight. Starving yourself is no good in the long run.
Instead, why not change a few of the foods you eat and the
way your cook them? While you are in a major change mode
you may as well get as much benefit in your life as you can.
If quality food costs a little more you can justify spending
some of the money you save on cigarettes.

Exercises for life

Better still, why not add an exercise regime to your new
non-smoking life? This has lots of advantages. It provides
the habits you will need to replace the smoking-related
habits you decide to drop. So you don't need to concoct
any. Exercise has its own benefits in addition to those you
will gain by becoming a non-smoker (see Harry Alder's
book *How to Live Longer*). Linking exercise with diet is a
proven formula for long life and well being. It doesn't need
to be a formal exercise regime. You can use the stairs
rather than lifts, walk or cycle on short journeys, do some
gardening or long-outstanding house repairs, or play with
the children. Do something with its own inherent benefits,
as that way – when applying it to stopping smoking – you

gain twice. The new habits associated with such a way of life will crowd out the old habits that have locked you into smoking dependence. The new sense of confidence you gain by mastering your smoking habits will stand you in good stead for these other beneficial lifestyle changes you want to make.

So you can turn this myth round into an opportunity:

- Replace cigarette dependence with a positive, all round healthier lifestyle.

- Put knowledge to use. Knowing that many smokers who give up put on a small amount of weight is a useful warning signal, and a logical reason to incorporate sensible eating and exercise into your new life.

- Instead of thinking of excuses to slowly poison yourself, think of excuses to introduce some beneficial habits into your life.

We have included these examples of smoking excuses because they are the most common. In practice, numerous attitudes and beliefs may affect how an individual copes with withdrawal. In most cases these are not easily identified as they do their work below the surface. In the next chapter you will learn how to understand yourself better, so that you can identify smoking-related beliefs and change them for more up-to-date, useful programmes.

(5)

Understanding Yourself

We run our lives according to mental programmes, or strategies – networks of electro-mechanical brain connections. These convert into words, feelings and behaviour, and operate with extraordinary efficiency and consistency. Unfortunately some get outdated, just like old software in your computer. We usually describe these programmes as **unwanted habits**. However, we rarely look upon unwanted habits as *positive* programmes, or intentions, because they usually conflict with what we consciously or rationally wish to do. Often we don't know why we act in certain ways.

At one time, however, such programmes fulfilled a useful purpose. For example, smoking as a teenager maybe helped you to fit in, be admired, or fulfil some such social need. Today such a strategy is not only no longer useful, but may be unconsciously thwarting your conscious attempts to give up the habit and live the way you want to live. The bottom line is that you can change these rogue programmes to suit your present needs and intentions. This includes any attitudes and beliefs about smoking that, as we have seen already, keep you locked into the habit. In this chapter we will concentrate on identifying what is going on inside, and understanding our-selves better. With this information you can then apply proven techniques to make the necessary **mind-programme changes**.

THE WEAKEST LINK

The problem with these mental programmes is that we don't always remember an old belief, so don't know it is there. You can't dump or print out the contents of a lifetime of brain data as you can the data on a hard disk. This applies to the old beliefs and motivations that you ran when you experienced that first cigarette. When trying to give up, smokers usually don't realise that such programmes are still there, as they operate 'below the surface' of our conscious mind. We don't need to give them thought to survive day by day, so they get missed. Like a computer operating system, they just run in the background. You don't think about them until something goes wrong.

The difficulty people experience when trying to give up smoking is mainly psychological, or in the mind. As we have seen, physical addiction to the drug nicotine is something quite specific and straightforward to treat. The difference with psychological factors is not so much that they are complex or difficult to tackle, but that we don't easily identify them, so they get missed and do their damage by default. Even if you identify habits connected with smoking, such as the kind in the previous chapter, and which thus form part of the problem, there may be other beliefs and habits you *don't* associate, and yet which

unconsciously support your smoking behaviour.
Unfortunately, any unidentified smoking-related habit is the
very psychological weak link that will cause you to give in
to a cigarette a few days, weeks or even months down the
line. In this book we are only interested in *lifetime*
withdrawal, so we treat this aspect of giving up as crucial to
success.

It starts with understanding yourself, and 'how you tick',
especially in relation to your smoking habit. This includes
understanding how your unconscious mind supports
behaviour that your conscious, rational mind would never
have entertained for a moment. Understanding yourself may
also take you back in time, to when you started smoking.
Most smokers would not even consider starting smoking
today, given what they now know, so clearly different beliefs
and motivations applied at the time they started.
Remarkable as it may seem, these old beliefs and attitudes
persist long after their sell-by date. The benefits they
'sought' for you in the light of your then knowledge and
experience no longer apply. Once you can identify these old
mental programmes, it is a straightforward job to replace
them with more appropriate ones. The techniques you will
use are almost 100 per cent effective, given:

• a sincere desire to change

• proper identification of the mental strategies, or
  programmes that need to be changed

- reasonable skill in applying them – which you can learn and practise anyway – such as being able to visualise clearly.

We spend most of our lives looking after the here and now, and rarely stop to question all the habitual, 'unthinking' behaviour that fills most of our lives. Indeed, if we behaved rationally we would doubtless never touch another cigarette. However, as with any habit, we act *without thinking*, or until it is too late. This applies to every one of us, and to all kinds of attitudes and behaviour. It just happens that the smoking habit is a particularly damaging one, so the *consequential* effect of an old habit is so much worse. Most smokers sincerely want to gain control over whatever causes their continued, slavish behaviour and understanding oneself is a vital part of the process.

ASKING WHY

In this chapter we will ask two crucial questions. Address these honestly and thoroughly and you immediately multiply your chances of permanent success.

1. Why did I start in the first place?

2. Why do I continue?

This is part of a self-understanding process that also includes the vital question that we covered in Chapter 3: what will I *give up* as a non-smoker?

Giving up involves *change*, which humans are not too keen on, and the important changes happen in the mind. There is nevertheless some *know-how*, or skill, involved in getting in touch with your subconscious mind in order to identify hidden motives and beliefs. Some people can do this more easily than others, but anybody can with a little practice (we all had super imaginations as children). It just comes down to getting into a relaxed state of mind in which busy, present-moment thoughts don't get the attention they usually do. This is the state of mind for daydreaming or just 'going inside', such as when on a long car drive, when we focus on other than our immediate surroundings. The only difference is that you now want to do this purposely, and in particular, to focus on the smoking issue.

Getting into the best state of mind for any kind of introspection calls mainly for common sense. For instance, find a comfortable place and choose a time when you are unlikely to be interrupted. Choose a place you associate with pleasure, and in which you can easily wind down, rather than somewhere such as an office with associations of stress or conflict. Otherwise simply relax as best you know how. Most people have their own methods, such as listening to calming music, choosing a comfortable chair, having a hot bath, waiting till the children are off to sleep and so on. If you don't have a method, the so-called countdown method, described opposite works for most people.

Countdown to control

As you count down from say 50 to one, progressively relax every part of your body. Start with your limbs and make them heavy (or light) one at a time. Use your imagination – make your legs lead or plaster of Paris, for instance, or helium-filled balloons. At the same time breathe deeply, slowly and rhythmically. Eventually every part of you will be physically relaxed, including your neck, facial muscles and eyes. While you are doing this you can visualise a pleasant environment – a special place, for instance, in which you feel safe, calm and confident. This may be a place from memory, enhanced as much as you like, or completely fantastic. Visualisation helps you to mentally relax and remove busy thoughts. In particular it excludes critical arguments from your conscious, left brain. With a little practice, you will be able to adapt the state quickly with a countdown of ten to one.

Having done the ten to one exercise a few times, you will have acquired the know-how to get into the necessary state of mind to carry out the self-understanding processes in this chapter. So before you go any further have a go, and ensure that you are happy about relaxing and visualising. Bear in mind that this core mental skill – the ability to relax any time and 'go inside' – will bring lots of other health and self-improvement benefits in addition to giving up smoking. We can now address the first question.

WHY DID I START IN THE FIRST PLACE?

The first thing you can be sure about is that there certainly was a reason, or several reasons, why you started to smoke. And we mean *reasons* – to you, that is – rather than excuses. Moreover, any reason must have then been a compelling one, because it takes a lot of determination to overcome the initial displeasure of smoking cigarettes, as it would ingesting any poison. It may be some years ago in your case, but you will need to take yourself back to the first occasion to recall it vividly. In this way you will be able not just to recall the unpleasant taste and symptoms of the cigarette, but also to get insight into why you persevered and in due course established smoking as a regular part of your life. You may find yourself pondering this question as you read.

Most smokers start as teenagers and the common factor seems to be peer pressure, but the initial stimulus may be more specific. It may be fear of offending or losing a particular friend, for instance, rather than not fitting into a group. Usually it involves a person's self-esteem, or feeling of worth. It may date to a specific dare, experiment or youthful rite of passage. Maybe you thought the practice would attract the attention of someone you wanted to notice you. Or it may have been a response to the advertising that created the illusion that smoking was 'cool' or 'grown up'. The point is that these constitute very real factors to a person at an impressionable age, with his or her knowledge and understanding.

Once the behaviour takes hold, after sufficient repetition, your unconscious mind establishes habits that run automatically. Further behaviour 'proves' to your unconscious mind – the behavioural 'control room' – that you are serious in your intentions, that you wanted it, that it is of value. That is, your behaviour was not an unintentional 'one off'. In doing so it doesn't apply logic, ethics or any rational criteria. It simply serves you in fulfilling your assumed desire – however short-sighted, immature or stupid. And – importantly for our present purposes – it will do so faithfully and for as long as that desire exists somewhere in your subconscious mind. Hence the fact that habits can be both good and bad, and in both cases powerful and self-fulfilling in that they reinforce themselves with time and practice.

Peer pressure probably does not tell the full story, and nor might the specific circumstances of that first cigarette. Certain *underlying causes* were strong enough to create the persistent behaviour – perhaps the need for attention, acceptance, friendship and so on. Such major, unarticulated motivations could probably have been fulfilled in other ways, but clearly smoking fulfilled the psychological need at the time.

Back to the beginning

You may already be forming reasons why you started. That's fine, but it is necessary to do the job thoroughly in a relaxed, 'downtime' mode. So follow the relaxation process on page 88, or use the system that works best for you, then take your mind back to that first cigarette and ask the following sorts of questions:

- Where were you?

- When did it happen?

- Who were you with?

- What were the circumstances just before?

- What did it taste like?

- What was your physical reaction?

- What else went through your mind?

- What benefits did it give?

- Were you proud of your behaviour or ashamed?

- Did you tell people close to you or hide it?

- Did you know then what you know now about the dangers of smoking?

- Might you have acted differently if you had known the danger?

- Are you wiser now?

- Do the same things motivate you as did when you smoked your first cigarette?

In a relaxed, trance-like state you will find your mind exploring the event and other things that happened at the time, and perhaps over the following days and weeks. It is as though you were re-living the actual experiences. You may recall circumstances and events that had never occurred to you. In particular, you may realise that you knew no better at the time, that your circumstances were very different, and how different your attitude is today. Write down the answers that come to mind. These form the basis of the strategies that your mind has run so successfully since that time. The same mentally-programmed strategies faithfully ensure your continued psychological dependence on smoking behaviour. Making a list will help you to accept that such mindsets or programmes exist. It will also serve as a checklist, which you will need to refer to when carrying out the change programmes in Chapter 6.

Having carried out this exercise you may indeed find that none of the reasons you identify, such as wanting to appear grown up, apply today. In this case you will be ready to immediately discard the old beliefs – and simply bringing them to the surface usually quashes their power over your behaviour. On the other hand, one or more reasons may still strike a chord. For example, you may still feel the need to fit into a particular social group, just as you did back then. Nonetheless, having honestly identified the reasons you are well on the way to a solution. In the next section you will address any such remaining reasons that might explain why you continue to smoke. You can now do this rationally as an adult, with the advantage of all the knowledge and experience you have gained over the years – as well as a better understanding of why you started in the first place.

WHY DO I CONTINUE?

You are now ready to think about your present situation. To understand why you continue to smoke, when all the facts argue to the contrary, you will need to follow more or less the same process. This time you need not delve back into distant memories, but you do need to get in touch with your unconscious mind, as this is clearly where the habit is being master-minded against your better judgement. Once again, try to identify any benefits or advantages you perceive from smoking. Consider also the disadvantages and harm, not just to your own health and wellbeing, but – if it matters to you – to other people. Sometimes the mental addiction is so powerful that we can overlook what would be the obvious feelings of other people and the harm we are doing to them as well as ourselves. This means, in effect, taking your head out of the sand and exposing yourself to the childlike frankness of your unconscious mind.

To answer the apparently simple question 'Why do I continue?' you will need to ask yourself more specific questions:

- What causes me to light up?

- In what situations do I usually want to smoke?

- What times and events during the day trigger a cigarette?

- What sort of feelings make me automatically resort to a cigarette?

- What changes in lifestyle would make it easier for me to resist the urge to smoke?

- What, specifically, do I get out of smoking?

- What is the best thing about cigarettes in my life?

- What is the worst thing about smoking?

- Do I sincerely want to give up?

- Are there any other factors that might affect my smoking or not smoking?

Again, write down your answers and thoughts. In a relaxed state of mind you will probably think of other insightful questions that will help specifically in your case.
It is especially important to establish what positive benefits you perceive that you now gain from smoking, for three reasons:

1. These perceptions may also turn out to be outdated 'programmes' that, upon honest appraisal, are no more valid than the reasons why you started to smoke.

2. They may be based on a misunderstanding of the association between the cigarette and other aspects of your life that give pleasure (or reduce pain) – such as a meal with friends, as we saw in the previous chapter.

3. You can only make changes once you can identify what needs to be changed.

Understanding yourself is important in many more aspects of your life than smoking, of course. Intrapersonal intelligence is a major constituent of so-called **emotional intelligence**, and is a factor in self development and personal and professional success generally. We are all more than capable of such self-awareness. But – as with a vivid imagination that many people seem to lose when passing from childhood to adulthood – we often need to practise and develop it as a mental skill. This includes basic relaxation and multi-sensory visualisation, and generally using your imagination. This is the know-how that complements the 'facts' or knowledge you need about smoking before you can give it up for certain. Few smokers go through this self understanding process and are quite unprepared for giving up – or at least staying that way. It doesn't take much intelligence to imagine the sort of situations in which one might give in to a cigarette after a day or two – most smokers have been through that experience. Nor does it require rocket science to prepare so that you minimise the risks. Even more importantly, only by identifying what is going on inside can you tackle the mental addiction that represents the lion's share of the smoker's problem.

By now you should have become familiar with visualisation as a tool, and have some answers to the important questions we have addressed in this chapter. You are ready to do some lifetime re-programming.

6

Programming Your Mind

What you think about most is most likely to happen. It turns into behaviour. That makes all kinds of change possible because you can think anything you like. We have already seen how we create behavioural programmes by default, and these account for habits such as smoking. You can adopt the same mind-body programming system more purposefully, for specific, positive goals. For example, you could visualise yourself as a non-smoker at a forthcoming work or social event, or in some context in which you would normally smoke. That sort of visualisation creates a **non-smoking programme**, which affects your unconscious, habitual behaviour. It reinforces your conscious mind that 'decides' to stop, and left-brain traits such as will, common sense and perseverance.

Many smokers use these 'right-brain' imagery techniques in other contexts of their life with great success. It is just a matter of applying them differently. If necessary, the simple relaxation and visualisation exercises in this chapter will furnish you with the necessary skills. Based on the old beliefs and attitudes to smoking you identified, you are now ready to create new strategies by changing these mental programmes once and for all.

Creating a new future

Visualising can do wonders when it comes to changing behaviour, and especially unwanted habits. I received a letter from Beth, a management trainee, several months after a seminar I conducted. She thanked me because she had given up smoking, and she described how it happened. She repeatedly visualised the forthcoming Christmas holiday with her friends and family as a non-smoker. She experienced all the compliments and sheer pleasure of not being a slave to her long-time habit. New tastes, smells and insignificant experiences came alive as long-lost pleasures. Christmas came and by then she was *actually* a non-smoker, experiencing just what she had repeatedly visualised.

Remarkably, she had felt no withdrawal symptoms whatsoever. In that sense it was a 'non-event', she said. She just became 'the way she saw herself' in her imagined new person. It was as natural and as simple as that. But the most remarkable aspect of this story to me was that the seminar was nothing to with giving up smoking, and I don't recall even raising the topic. It was to do with the power of visualisation to create a new future, and that was the principle she took away and used to such powerful effect. You can change by clearly visualising what you want to do and be. Vivid visualisation harnesses your imagination and gets right to the source, or control centre, of the behaviour you want to change.

USING YOUR WHOLE BRAIN

To make changes to old programmes you will need to 'go inside', just as you did when identifying the reasons why you started to smoke, and continue to do so. As we saw in the previous chapter, to do that you had to imagine, or visualise, the past and the present – such as situations in which you automatically reach for a cigarette. The same principles apply when creating the new programmes: the better you can relax, get into a 'downtime' mode and visualise clearly, the more effective the change process.

Whatever knowledge you amass, this is important *know-how*, and part of the preparation for giving up once and for all. Most readers will find the process easy, as we all use our imagination in different aspects of our lives. If you have difficulty, it is worth practising before you commit yourself to a definite decision to quit. You can do just about anything with practice, including mental activities such as visualisation and self-hypnosis. Moreover, if you can do something once – like vividly reliving your first day at a new school, or a memorable childhood event, or winning an accolade in a sport or pastime you enjoy – you can repeat it *in other situations*. Better still, it gets easier with each attempt and has a disproportionately greater effect on your behaviour. It soon becomes a habit – the easiest kind of behaviour. Mastering this fundamental 'skill' is a wise investment of your time. You will call upon it at each stage in the process, and long after you have smoked your last cigarette. As an added bonus, it applies to other kinds of self-development and change.

Mental programming is more than invisible, ethereal 'software'. That's a fine metaphor as far as it goes. However, in fact the human brain *physically* creates new, electro-chemical, neural networks as we think, reflect and imagine. That means you don't need to *pretend* when you use these mental skills: you will *become* what you visualise – in this case the healthy new person you want to be, with habits that you choose rather than habits that seem to choose you.

Imagination and willpower

Visualising is a good example of a right-brain activity, and it is true to say that many of the important changes happen there. In this case it is not an act of the will, but of the imagination. Or not so much of the mind as the heart. However, as well as visualising, or imagining, we use our mind in a quite logical, cerebral or 'left brain' way. We do this when we make a firm decision to do or not do something. It's called willpower.

In fact willpower *alone* may not be enough to change a longstanding habit, as many long-term smokers know only too well, but this doesn't mean you don't require an act of will. You certainly do, and this applies also to dieting and just about any other habitual behaviour you want to change. Fortunately, as humans, we can all exercise will or purpose: you decide to do something, then do it. It is not so much willpower as intention. You focus your intention by giving it your attention. Or, as a simple formula:

I + fa + a = M (Intention + focused attention + action = Manifestation).

When handled in a step-by-step way, rational changes of this sort are quick and easy. When directed towards what you want, rather than what you don't want, they can also be pleasurable.

The bottom line is that you need to use your *whole brain* when making lifetime changes – heart and mind, right brain and left brain, intuition and common sense. Your whole brain runs the show as a smoker, and only your whole brain can run the show as a non-smoker. It should now be obvious why most people repeatedly fail to properly give up their 'habit', leaving so much software untouched, and beliefs and behaviour unchanged. You can learn from their experience.

Change techniques

In Chapter 5 you used visualisation to help identify the old smoking programmes. We visualise a past experience, for instance, in the form of a memory. You also used visualisation to help get into a relaxed, or downtime mode. This is when the brain ticks over at a slow frequency. It is the hypnotic, or trance state in which we are most amenable to suggestion and literal changes of mind. In these cases, visualisation helps to identify beliefs and thinking patterns that need to be changed, but it is also important when making actual changes. It works according to a very simple principle:

- The human brain does not know the difference between an external sensory reality, and a clearly visualised imagination.

This is best illustrated in dreaming. You wake from a vivid
dream and for a few moments you don't know whether you
are in the dream or the real world. In fact, it is one and the
same world inside – a world we create through a complex
brain network of synaptic 'firings'. That's our only world as
individuals. Visualisation gives you a fast track route into
this personal inner world, and a vehicle for changing it.

The idea occurs in philosophy and religion also, in the
sense that 'Whatever a man thinks, so he is'. As we said
earlier, you are (or will become) what you think about
most. Thus everything in the man-made world was first a
visualised or imagined reality, before we transformed it (by
behaviour) into external 'reality.' This sets human
imagination in a most powerful light, and highlights the
importance of mental imagery in making the sort of life
changes we are concerned with. Giving up smoking
involves more than thinking about it, of course. It involves
behaviour, but behaviour starts in the mind, and it is in
the mind that you need to take control of it.

Using your imagination is the best sort of change technique
as it is so natural. You don't need drugs and there are no
detrimental side effects. It is what children do when they
want something badly. They dream about it so much until it
is as real as a 'real' imaginary friend. If they want a bike,
they will scan the colour brochures, drag their parents to
the store, think about it, dream about it, touch it and feel it
in their imagination and all but own the thing. More often
than not, come Christmas or a timely birthday, the bike

101

becomes a reality. And if cynical parents think this is just their way to an easy life, the same principle applies in career planning, entrepreneurship, political ambition, dreams of foreign travel, sporting aspirations and so on. Successful people live their lives backwards – they 'create' a future in their mind and start to live *into* that future.

* Visualising a successful future is an established principle of human achievement and change.

So here is an easy route to changing smoking habits. It concerns not just what you do, but who and what you are. That is, the change to becoming a non-smoker. The skill or know-how covers two areas:

1. Mental skill
First is the skill in actual visualisation, and that applies to visualising for *any* purpose (you can use it in many aspects of your life). This involves using all five senses to the full. For instance, in the case of seeing you can explore focus, brightness, colour, distance, dimension, movement and so on. In the case of hearing you may notice the volume, timbre, tone, rhythm, continuity and so on. The more you explore the mental characteristics (or submodalities) of an experience, the more real it becomes, simply because real life is rich and varied in just this way. So multi-sensory visualisation is like adding to real life experience, but without recourse to the outside world with its mistakes and disappointments. You can create or change mental programmes, just as you do as you experience new

sensations day by day. The result is *habitual* behaviour. It becomes easy – just as when you conscientiously practise any simple activity in real life.

2. Choosing what you want
The second area concerns the *subject* you visualise, and the way you represent it. An important rule in this case is to imagine what you *want* rather than what you *don't* want. Most people focus on the very things they *don't* want. In golf, for instance, instead of visualising the tree, bunker or water hazard you want to avoid, you need to visualise the hole you want to reach or a particular spot on the fairway. In other words, think about what you want to *hit* rather than what you want to *miss*. This simple change of mental perspective will revolutionise a person's game. The same principle applies not just to any sport, but to any human behaviour, including quitting smoking. It means seeing yourself as a healthy, non-dependent person in every respect – rather than concentrating on either the unpleasant consequences of smoking, the difficulties of withdrawing or the image of failure. You visualise instead your desired state, or future.

Imagining what you don't want is sometimes called worry, which tends to be self-fulfilling – much like the proverbial 'accident waiting to happen'. 'Negative visualisation' is also associated with pessimism, and research has established that optimistic thinkers outperform pessimists in actual life achievement several times over. Hence the importance not just of the technique, at which inveterate worriers are masters, but of the attitude and perspective you take.

Notice that even though our attitude affects actual behaviour, it all happens in the mind. The vital need is therefore to change the mental programmes you run, rather than trying to change the outward, visible behaviour they produce. That is why willpower alone – to almost any level – will not change a well-established habit.

In the case of giving up smoking, Beth (see page 87) focused on becoming the person she wanted to be, rather than the downsides of being the smoker she decided she didn't want to be. Specifically, she did not imagine giving up (the process) but what it would be like to have already given up (the new person and new behaviour). Metaphorically, she looked to the destination rather than the journey. If we had a positive word for non-smoker, she visualised being one.

Using your imagination

Although the concept is simple, creating the future you want calls for some ingenuity. For instance, you can imagine not just the obvious consequences of being a non-smoker, but the less obvious spin-off benefits. For example, as well as visualising in detail the differences at home with your family, you would explore many work and social situations, or situations that don't occur every day or week, yet are important in your life – such as Christmas, holidays, annual events, periodic family reunions and so on. In fact, these are often the very occasions when a smoker relapses. By incorporating them into your mental preparation, they become a resource, or opportunity for visualisation – a foundation, if you like, for your mental programme. At the same time, when the occasion arises, even though you may still experience the temptation, you will intuitively use your well-rehearsed new behaviour rather than allow the old mental programme to do its work. In addition, the benefits you envisage add to your motivation (just like a child wanting a new bike, you want it more and more) and change your attitudes and beliefs about smoking. You now have more empowering programmes to run your life.

The deeper (in quality and richness) and wider (in situations, such as at work and socially) you can apply visualisation, the more like multi-dimensional real life your internal image will become. Each new benefit you explore will add to your motivation as you are drawn towards the good things you imagine. Motivation is at the core of any important life change, and usually means the difference between success and failure – whether winning an Olympic medal, overcoming a physical handicap, or changing an unwanted behaviour. This includes the important life change in becoming a non-smoker. So explore in your imagination the pleasure and benefits of being the free, healthy person you want to be.

BELIEF AND BEHAVIOUR

As we have seen, mental programmes, or strategies, control all your behaviour. It works the other way too. What you do affects your mind – the way you feel, your attitude, motivation and so on. How many times have we fought off a black cloud of depression by getting on with some physical activity at work, or clearing out the garage or cupboards at home? In other words, *acting* differently. We

whistle when we are happy, but we become happier when we
whistle. This is a feature of the holistic nature of the human
'body-mind' system. As we saw earlier, it's all one system –
body and mind are interdependent.

This offers us another valuable principle that we can use
when changing old smoking-related beliefs. Remember the
split-brain experiments? The subjects' belief was affected by
what they actually witnessed – in other words, by actual
behaviour. This applies universally. For example, you can
believe you are a loser in a sport, but if you have a string of
wins it becomes more and more difficult to sustain your
loser belief. Or you can believe you don't have confidence,
but if you find you are *acting* confidently over a period you
will have to reconsider your self-belief. In short, we can
utilise the effect of belief on behaviour, but we can also
utilise the powerful effect of behaviour on belief, including
the beliefs that sustain the smoking habit. Specifically, you
may believe you are a smoker, but if your mind records non-
smoker-type behaviour, you have to start believing
differently – and that breaks the vicious circle.

In real life this principle presents a problem of the chicken
and egg sort. What are the chances of *acting* confidently if
your belief system militates against it and – as we have seen
– controls your behaviour in the first place? What are the
chances of acting like a non-smoker if you can hardly last
out for an hour? The answer is to *work the system*, and
carry out the behaviour *inside*, by visualisation. This
combines two principles we met earlier:

1. Acting out your self-belief and identity reinforces those mental programmes – the 'whistle to be happy' principle.

2. The brain does not know the difference between reality and a clearly envisaged behaviour.

In short, successful behaviour *inside* has the same effect as successful behaviour *outside*. More than that, *repeated* internal behaviour has the same effect as *repeated* external behaviour. Practice makes perfect, including mental practice, and the more practice the more perfect.

The role of mental practice

There is more to it, and this makes visualisation the powerful tool it is. There are three important differences between mental practice and practice in real life:

1. In real life we 'miss' as often, or more often, as we 'hit'. In the case of putting in golf, for example, we fail *far* more times than we succeed. In trying to give up smoking, we fail far more often than we succeed – in effect, having decided we want to give up, every time we light up. So we *practise failure* rather than success – and get better at failing! Hence the ever-tightening grip of the smoking habit. That is why wilfully cutting down by clocking up a few successes a day can have a counterproductive result – the habit continues to be reinforced, by 'failure practice', at a greater level.

2. Real life practice takes time and can be hard work. However, you can visualise your mental programme

changes from an armchair. This is not psychobabble. Research involving basketball free throws showed a significant improvement in overall level of performance simply by using mental practice! It was very close to the improvement in a group that practised physically for the same period each day. This makes mental practice:

- easy – you can do it in your armchair
- efficient – in time and effort
- and effective – it simulates real life and brings about actual changes in habits.

3. You can speed up processes mentally. You can, for instance, practise scores of activities, such as a sports stroke or shot, in the time it would take to do just one in real life – and that ignores the drive in the rain to the gym, football pitch or wherever. An extreme, but graphic example of this speeding up phenomenon is when a person sees their life 'passing before them' in the moments during which they think they are about to die. You don't need anything like that speed to accumulate scores of successful 'experiences' as a non-smoker, but it is a mental skill worth harnessing for your purposes. We utilise this mental phenomenon whenever we quickly imagine a whole future scenario.

All these mental characteristics provide very useful devices for changing behaviour. It means that even if a visualised image is far less real than a 'real' image (say 50 per cent for argument's sake), the fact that you only mentally practise success rather than failure more than makes up the difference. In other words, what you might lose in realism, you can more than make up for in sheer volume of 'success recordings'. You don't waste mental energy. Similarly, by speeding up the process you can again more than make up the difference. This doesn't take effort – we normally think a lot faster than we behave outwardly anyway. On the contrary, imagining what you really want, and all the pleasure that goes with it, is rather like enjoying the anticipation of a well-deserved holiday as much as the holiday itself.

You may initially want to establish a regular routine of positive visualisation – say first thing in the morning, then at a regular, convenient time during your day, then again last thing before going to sleep when your brain is in a very receptive state. However, once you learn to use the technique effectively, you can increase your chances of success as much as you wish. You now have the knowledge and know-how, and that means control.

You can even visualise an apparent failure, as well as always finishing up on top. For example, see yourself being offered a cigarette, putting it to your mouth, realising how disgusting it appears and calmly stubbing it out. This is a sort of programmed safety net.

- Do not underestimate the power of simple mental rehearsal.

People have won medals, amassed fortunes and attained the highest positions in society on the basis of a repeated, clearly visualised dream. It's not overkill to apply these natural mental processes to a life-changing switch to being the person you want to be. The person you want to be must first be born in your mind.

CHANGING BELIEFS

We can now incorporate all this into a simple belief change process. This builds on everything that you have read in the book so far. That includes not just the specific techniques in the previous chapter for identifying smoking-related mind programmes, but also the earlier facts and arguments that work on your mind unconsciously and incrementally. If you skipped any of this and want to read on with a view to working through the book more carefully, that's fine. It will have a greater effect second time through anyway. Otherwise you are likely to have missed an important link in the chain that will do its unwanted job two days – or six months – after you quit. If you really intend to go through with giving up permanently you may as well do the job properly and not pretend that you are somehow different from other people and can control psychological phenomena that you may not even be aware of. That's why we chose the title of the book.

Beliefs are not 'real', of course, they are constructed in our minds. That means we can deconstruct them to support the behaviour we prefer, once we know how. So here is the belief change process:

1. Write down all the things you will believe about your new self as a non-smoker. These replace the old beliefs you identified that made sense when you started, but no longer apply. For example:

- I am relaxed in company, such as after a meal, with no artificial props whatsoever.

- I can easily concentrate and focus my mind when I need to.

- I am accepted for who I am by friends and colleagues. I don't need to pretend.

Add as many as you can think of that reflect your unique situation. By writing them down and saying them out loud you are stating clearly your new beliefs, and creating the programmes that will run your behaviour as a non-smoker.

2. Think of three examples of behaviour that will illustrate or support these beliefs. For example, imagine different situations in which you are completely relaxed and in control, yet with not a cigarette in sight, or situations at work or at home when you can concentrate for as long as you wish without drugs or props of any kind. As you live out the behaviour clearly state your belief. Why three? Make it 33 if you like, but you need to convince your unconscious mind that you are really a different person and that the old beliefs are no longer true. We saw earlier the effect of repetition in creating habits, but this process does something more. Compare it with a person who is confident in many different aspects of their life – at work, at home, socially, in adversity, when provoked and so on. Each different demonstration of their confidence adds to their deep belief and identity as a 'confident person'. A person who is only confident in one or two areas (such as a sport or hobby) often does

not see him- or herself as a confident *person*. Put another way, this will programme not just what you *do* as a non-smoker, but what you *are*. It forms a high-level 'meta programme' that will stand the test of time, and run a whole battery of different behaviour to support it.

3. Add to this effect by making your visualised examples more and more vivid or true to life. As a checklist use not just the five senses – in your imagining see, hear, feel, and smell and taste if applicable, but also the sorts of qualities we suggested earlier: For example, make your pictures bigger and brighter, and turn up the volume if you wish. Experiment with these qualities with a view to intensifying the experience, which strengthens the new belief programme. It is a matter of mental credibility. We are not convinced by a poor painting or badly acted television drama and the test is often whether we are drawn into the picture or story because it is 'true to life'. Vivid, multi-sensory mental imagery is *credible*, just as though you had represented the 'real' outside world. The new programme therefore has the same power as the repeated behaviour that forms any habit, including the repeated smoking that originally convinced your unconscious mind that you were now a real McCoy smoker whether by 'addiction' or wilful perseverance under social pressure. You can tap into the same behaviour-creating system.

4. Repeat your visualised belief-supporting behaviours, again as many times as you care to. Remember that you have mentally and physically rehearsed the old behaviour maybe thousands of times throughout your

period as a smoker, and this process helps to redress the balance. Fortunately, recent memories have a greater effect than old ones, so your repeated, *accelerated* visualisation over the few days before finally quitting can counterbalance years of the old smoking habits.

Don't look on this exercise as a chore. Beth, the management trainee, who gave up before Christmas (page 87), enjoyed every minute of her imagined new life before it ever happened.

Now, as well as declaring your new belief, you have backed it up in practice, based on the established principle that your brain does not differentiate between clearly visualised imagery and reality. You became a smoker inside first (the image of the cool, grown up person you wanted to be), then outside next. Likewise, you will become a non smoker inside first, and outside next. As you practise internally by mental rehearsal, or visualisation, you will establish true habits to replace those you don't want. And all this mental practice adds to your motivation – the key to giving up for good.

RECONCILING 'PARTS'
Because of the conflict between our conscious and unconscious mind it seems as if there are different parts to us. The rational, conscious part wants to do one thing, while another part of us – a very powerful part – seems bent on doing something else. This latter part clearly operates below our conscious level. It is responsible for the reflex-type habits that perpetuate smoking, the beliefs or mental

113

strategies that sustain them, and consequently the difficulties in giving up.

Understanding the characteristics of how we think as parts offers us an opportunity when it comes to smoking cessation. One part wants to carry on smoking while the other part wants to stop – and somehow the latter part hasn't had its proper say. These parts represent high-level or **meta programmes** that control your identity as a smoker. Change at this level will affect every nuance of your behaviour. As with the approach to changing beliefs we have just met, it just means knowing and harnessing the system. In this case you can carry out a simple exercise that *reconciles* the two parts – the part of you that wants to carry on smoking, and the part of you that wants to stop. Do this exercise in a relaxed, downtime, trancelike state in the way you should now be familiar with.

'Parts' exercise

1. When fully relaxed, imagine each part of you is in a separate hand. You can hold your hands out, palms up, if you wish. Name the two parts so that you know which is which (such as the judge and the gremlin – but use your own labels). Consider one part, and think about its feelings, fears, hopes and beliefs. Write down each of its concerns, regarding its behaviour, what is important, how it feels and so on. What does it want? What does it not want? Especially let it express how it feels about the other part in a non-judgemental way, ready to understand why the other part feels and acts as it does.

The old smoking beliefs you have already identified will
provide a checklist.

2. Do the same with the other part. Stop writing for a
    while to allow your mind to go deep and really
    communicate with your inner self, but get the points
    down on paper at some point so that you can refer back
    to them. Be frank and fair with both parts – let them
    have their say. Especially, what is the *positive intention*
    of the part that still wants to smoke?

Initially you may only *identify*, rather than reconcile the
issues, or come to a mutual decision, but that is a good
start. Go back to each part in turn and let them respond to
the arguments made by the other part, then if anything
remains unresolved do this again. Let each part express its
point of view fully and without criticism. The smoker part
might reveal reasons that go back several years. These may
now seem more reasonable in the light of what you knew
then and the social pressures and influences on your life.
At the time, this part of you sought to look after your
interests as best it knew. Usually an informed, 'adult'
perspective dissolves any real difference and brings the
parts together, just like making up with a friend after a
long period of alienation.

You may well find that some of the parts' concerns relate
back to the reasons you *started* smoking, rather than the
current reasons. Each part can now understand this with its
present, combined, *communicated* knowledge. It is as if a
severed connection between two parts of your brain were

joined up again. You need not be critical, and indeed you can thank your 'gremlin' for seeking – in the best way it knew how – to look after your interests. In most cases, once the parts are exposed to your conscious, rational mind the conflict will end.

With this new insight you will no longer wonder why you act out of character. Instead – if a smoking action is about to happen – you will *notice* it, understand what is happening and do something about it. As you regain conscious control, the old behaviour will lose its power. You have reprogrammed both parts to support your present, rather than past, intentions. The important revelation will be that both parts, at a higher level, want *the same thing* – to be a relaxed, confident, healthy, non-smoking person – and will readily agree on the non-smoking behaviour needed to achieve it. Once the parts start to work in the same direction you are well on the way to success.

Use this parts exercise in combination with the belief change exercise earlier. You may discover an old belief part of you of which you were not aware. You can then create a new belief to replace it, and visualise behaviour in three different situations to live out your new belief. Likewise, you can treat your 'old' and 'new' beliefs you identified as reflecting parts of you, and take account of them in the parts exercise.

YES OR NO
Affirmation is a well-proven technique for changing behaviour. You may have heard of Emile Coué's daily

affirmation 'Day by day, in every way, I'm getting better and better'. Affirmation means, in effect, saying 'yes' to what you want, and 'no' to whatever does not meet your desires. The strength of your 'yes' or 'no' will indicate the strength of a belief, value or mental programme. For example, some people can say 'no' to food while others say 'yes' all too easily. In extreme situations this will result in psychosomatic conditions such as anorexia, which illustrates the power of a belief like 'I'm fat' and its extreme effect on behaviour. Being psychologically addicted to smoking means, in effect, that you cannot say 'no' – or at least not resolutely enough. You can usually tell the degree of resolution by the way a person says 'yes' or 'no', and through their body language. To be sure of success, you need to learn to say 'no' to smoking behaviour and old mindsets, and 'yes' to the new behaviour and the new non-smoking person you will become.

The NLP (neuro linguistic programming) writer Michael Hall uses the term 'meta yes-ing', and 'meta no-ing'. 'Meta' refers to beliefs or values that happen at a higher level (meta = beyond) than most of our habitual behaviour. For example, the sensory changes in an earlier technique will affect much behaviour, but at the level of visualised sights, sounds and so on – whereas some of our behaviour is controlled at a higher 'logical' level of the mind. At this level lie beliefs, values and identity, which are more abstract, and affect the person holistically rather than at a specific activity level. The important point is that changes to so-called meta programmes will affect our behaviour – we act out what we think – but the reverse will not necessarily be the case. So just doing something differently will not of itself change your beliefs about yourself or your identity, for example as a smoker or non-smoker. Even if you stop smoking, your smoker identity will live on, and you will probably soon relapse.

- Change of this sort happens at a higher mental level – in the control centre rather than at the coal face.

Hence in the previous exercise we addressed the 'part' of you that identifies with the smoker in you, rather than the outward behaviour itself. The outward smoking behaviour – including indirect or associated behaviour – is a slave to controlling meta programmes. Conversely, by changing a meta programme you can now be master of a whole range of smoking-related behaviour.

We all know how to say 'yes' and 'no' in a way that will affect our behaviour. Think about something you would never entertain – something completely contrary to your values. Your reaction might be 'never, in no way, it's not negotiable' or suchlike. That reaction is your effective strategy for that belief, type of behaviour or aspect of your life. And it works. All your behaviour corresponds to that unequivocal mental programme. There is evidence of congruence between what you say (no) and what you do – your body language, tone of voice, and suchlike tends to match the words you use. Moreover, the programme is personal and 'learnt'. You weren't born with it. Indeed, you may know people with a very different point of view who would give an equally emphatic 'no' (or 'yes') to something they espouse strongly. The trick is to identify and utilise your own, proven motivation strategies.

Running your 'no' programme
By identifying your effective 'no' strategy, you can use it to give up smoking. Notice how you feel when you say it. What sensory experience can you recall? Imagine a circumstance in which you had to assert your 'no', and do a checklist of each sensory characteristic, such as size, colour and loudness – especially the feelings, or kinaesthetic sense. And how did you actually say 'no'? What tone, pitch and volume? In other words, what sort of 'no' to you *really* means 'no'?

This is invaluable self-knowledge, or intra-personal intelligence. It is the very 'no' you need to say to those smoking habits and another key to quitting. Start saying it, out loud when appropriate, but in any case repeatedly in your mind. As you do this, re-experience what you experienced when recalling your chosen example of a meta 'no' programme – the 'no' that has worked for you. Then utilise your 'no' resource for your specific intention to quit smoking.

Running your 'yes' programme
Apply the same technique to say 'yes' to the new non-smoker beliefs and behaviour you replaced the old ones with earlier. Once again, call upon your memory resources to find a good 'yes' programme. This time choose something you positively believe with every fibre of your being and that you reflect congruently in all your behaviour. In this case you

would normally answer equally emphatically, 'absolutely', 'no doubt whatsoever', '*yes*'. 'Do I love my children? Yes, of course I do.' Choose that sort of unequivocal affirmation, and again 'go inside' to identify and intensify the various sensory characteristics of what you recall, just as with the 'no' response.

Repeat your 'yes' often so that it becomes not just a deeply held belief or value, but an up-front, conscious affirmation that itself becomes a habit. With a little practice you will soon be able to instantly engage that committed 'yes' feeling, and use it whenever you need to. This will reinforce your belief in the new, non-smoking 'you' any time you feel you are slipping and negative messages enter your mind. It is a vital part of your preparation.

The power of meta programmes

Meta-yes-ing and no-ing takes a bit of practice, but it is a skill resource worth cultivating. Imagine all the other situations in which you can overcome unwanted behaviour using the same method. Simply utilise your proven, 'winning' mental strategy in the smoking part of your life in any area in which you badly need a 'win'.

As we have seen, mental programmes operate at different levels. One programme reaches for a cigarette according to a certain trigger or signal. A programme that says 'I am a smoker' works at a high level, and controls not just actual smoking behaviour, but also any smoking-related attitudes and beliefs that would not exist in the life of a non-smoker.

As we have seen, it is usually futile to tackle smoking behaviour if your identity remains as a smoker rather than a non-smoker. Hence the need to change the beliefs, or meta programmes, we have covered in this chapter.

PROGRAMMING BEHAVIOUR

Mental programmes determine our beliefs and attitudes, and what makes us tick as individuals, and lasting change has to happen at this level of the mind. The other side of the change coin is **actual behaviour**. In a technical sense, every behaviour down to micro-muscular level (apart from true reflex movements) requires an 'instruction' from the brain. But we are usually only *aware*, if we stop and think, of doing something *physically* – or externally – such as raising an arm, walking across the room, or taking a cigarette from the pack. It is therefore simpler to treat this aspect of smoking as physical. In this light, simple physical movements, of the sort associated with smoking, are as easy to do or not do, using will power, as any mental activity such as visualising the future or remembering the past. The only requirement is to think about what you are about to do – in other words *act consciously*. Once you can break the unconscious stimulus-response, you are free to carry out or not carry out basic 'smoking' actions.

Where then does the smoking problem arise? It reflects the mind-body system: once behaviour is established as a habit (and maybe 90 per cent of all our behaviour fits into this category) we do it *without thinking* – at least thinking in a conscious sense. The fact is we don't *need* to think, or do anything consciously. Hence we can walk and feed ourselves very efficiently, while thinking about *other* things at the same time; drive the car while listening to the radio and sorting out the children. And therein lies the problem. As well as carrying out sensible habits like climbing stairs, getting washed and opening the garage door, we get stuck with unwanted behaviours like steering the car with one hand, eating too much chocolate when we are worried, and *smoking*.

Thus setting up empowering meta programmes can also help to reprogramme specific activities or behaviour. This may not change a belief, but it will support and strengthen a belief (as with the three behaviours in the belief change exercise). Reprogramming applies especially in stimulus-response type behaviour. For example, the telephone rings at work and you light up. You set off walking for the train in the morning and automatically light up. You finish your meal in a restaurant and automatically light up, and so on. These are the habitual associations that, together, lock you into a total smoking habit and make quitting a far bigger problem than the addictive characteristics we met earlier can ever account for. In such cases you can specifically reprogramme your behaviour to respond differently. The stimuli will continue, of course – the telephone will still ring and you will continue to set out for work in the morning. But you can *condition* yourself to act differently just as at some point in the past you conditioned yourself (unknowingly, by practice and repetition) to your present stimulus-response smoking behaviour. You were not born a smoker – you had to learn the behaviour. So you *unlearn* it.

The swish method

The so-called swish method fits the bill in this case. See two pictures of yourself. The first is the picture you see when acting out the unwanted, smoking behaviour you want to change. Choose the moment *just before* you would normally act out the smoking behaviour – that is, the moment the trigger or stimulus occurs. That's the moment in real life when you now want to act differently as a non-smoker. Make the image what you see with your own eyes, and feel, rather than as an observer. For example, you may see your hand reaching for a cigarette as you move towards the telephone, see your friends across the restaurant table as you reach in your pocket for a packet, see a colleague lighting up and so on.

In the second picture, see yourself enacting the behaviour you would prefer. Make this compelling, by making things bigger, brighter, more attractive and more realistic. Use your ingenuity when deciding on suitable replacement behaviour. You might see yourself looking super confident, perhaps with a fancy new fountain pen in your cigarette hand (give yourself rewards), or sipping a fruit juice (drink plenty of fluid when withdrawing), or however you would prefer to occupy your hands. You will have super white teeth, stain-free fingers and sweet-smelling breath, of course. Choose any activity, posture or disposition you like instead of the unwanted nicotine habit. Don't just see yourself *doing* this, but *be* it – act out the full non-smoker role. Enjoy the benefits you identified earlier.

In this second picture, see yourself as if from outside, rather than through your own eyes. That image will be particularly motivating and draw you unconsciously towards it, just as a budding Olympic medallist sees him- or herself standing on the victory podium. Make these images clear and familiar enough by practice so that you can instantly see one or the other.

Next make the attractive, replacement image very small, like a postage stamp or even a dot, and place it in the bottom corner of the unwanted, 'trigger' picture. Then rapidly make the dot engulf the whole unwanted image in an instant, so that now *it* becomes the dot. Do this repeatedly – replacing the old image with the new just like an expanding airbag – getting faster and faster with each 'swish'. In between dot-to-full-picture switches, open your eyes and blank your mind completely from the images – spell your name backwards, count up in sevens, or do anything that will clear your mind. Do the 'swish' a dozen or so times, making the actual change as fast as possible – less than a second – while maintaining the vividness of the pictures. In that way, when in real life you are confronted with the realistic trigger image, the replacement picture will not just automatically appear but will motivate you.

Speed is vital. It confuses the old brain programme, and at the same time it will anchor the trigger to the new picture and therefore stimulate the response you want. You can say 'whoosh' or 'swish' once each time you do it. From now on it will not be possible to see the old trigger image without the new one swishing it out. Try it. Then try it again tomorrow. If you need to, rehearse the process a few more times. Usually the swish programme will remain effective for weeks and certainly days, covering the important withdrawal period. Apply the swish method to each stimulus or smoking-related habit you identify. Even one automatic behaviour might be the cause of a relapse.

You can test this technique any time you like by **future pacing**, or visualising. Think of an actual, forthcoming situation in which the 'stimulus' picture would appear and you would have normally acted out the old smoking behaviour. Notice that you no longer have the same desire to smoke, and behave differently – you are now the new you.

• Imagined behaviour happens.

You can do this future pace first thing in the morning, for instance, so that you are confident that your new programme is working fine. In any event, now that you know the technique, you can repeat it whenever you wish to reinforce your new programme.

As we saw earlier, with enough repetition of any activity you will become as familiar with the new behaviour as you were with the old. And just as a new pathway through a forest soon replaces the old one as it gradually becomes overgrown, so your new habits will imperceptibly and naturally replace the old one. Indeed, you will acquire the new habit as easily as you have acquired the hundreds of other habits that fill your life.

7

Making a Permanent Break

The final break stage is straightforward: don't put any more cigarettes in your mouth. However, to be sure of success the three requirements are:

1. information
2. preparation and
3. motivation.

Information means more than the harrowing facts about smoking-related diseases. It includes information about yourself – including what makes you smoke, why you find it hard to stop and specifically why you may have failed in the past. It includes information about the process of giving up, and what will happen from that point in time. It includes information about how to reprogramme your mind to do what you want to do as a non-smoker.

Preparation includes getting all this information, of course, so the two requirements overlap.

Likewise, motivation started before you picked up the book, and grows as you gain vital knowledge, so this also spans the whole cessation process.

Preparation and motivation have special significance when it comes to making the final break, and in the period immediately following. In this final chapter, before explaining how to make the final break in a way that maximises your chances of success, we will address these two important requirements.

PREPARATION

Hardly any smoker succeeds – at least for more than a short period – when they stop on a whim, without thought and planning, and a *reason*. The 'whim', in fact, often reflects an underlying cause such as a change of circumstances, a comment taken to heart, or any sort of shock. It's better if you identify this and prepare accordingly.

Everything you have read so far is there to ensure you are fully prepared. Until you are ready – which means you *feel* ready, confident and raring to go – it is pointless to stop smoking as you are unlikely to succeed. Before long, after a further period of frustration or depression, you will probably want to go through it all again. But you will then have even more stress, and less confidence of success because of another failure.

Preparation need not be a gruelling, boring phase. We have already seen how pleasurable visualisation exercises can be – it's like enjoying a down payment, or a taste of all the benefits of being healthy, free and in control of your life. At the same time, as you change your beliefs and the strategies that run your behaviour, you may find that you are smoking less without trying, or even deciding on a date, so the benefits are not all in the mind. This will especially be the case after doing the swish exercises, which can change behaviour immediately. You become *aware* of the smoking 'trigger' situations you imagined whenever they arise, whereas previously you would have responded to them automatically – becoming 'aware' halfway through a cigarette, or when the ash tray had filled up – in other words, when it's too late.

- Having now **anchored** the replacement behaviour that you practised and tested, it will soon become the 'natural' thing to do.

- Combined with the different **attitude** you have to smoking due to the belief change programmes, and 'yes' and 'no' affirmations, smoking loses its attraction, and you start to smoke less.

Cutting down on cigarettes in this natural way is fine, as it happens from the inside out – or according to new mental strategies. Having prepared by changing your mental strategies, you don't need to rely on willpower to change your behaviour 'from the outside'. The test is that you hardly realise the change is happening, which is just the way habits should change. Beth, the lady who visualised herself as a non-smoker at the forthcoming Christmas, felt she was a non-smoker long before Christmas arrived, and found herself simply not wanting cigarettes. In other words, she started to act like a non-smoker. By the time she got to smoke her last cigarette, giving up was not an issue, as the new habits had been doing their subconscious job without fanfare.

MOTIVATION

In the book we have emphasised the importance of motivation – truly wanting to quit. Motivation often arises from circumstances in your life, such as an illness, a bereavement among family or friends caused through smoking, a shock, or something that brings you to a point of decision. Often something prompts a person to buy a book like this in the first place, and that may be the crucial turning point in their motivation. All your preparation so far, as well as providing information and skills, has been to increase your desire and commitment, up to the moment at which you make the final break and beyond.

Motivation increases in three ways during this preparation process:

1. The more reasons you have not to smoke, the more you want to give it up and change once and for all. This is the human tendency to move away from perceived pain and harm of any kind.

2. The more pleasure and benefits you can imagine as a non-smoker, the more you will be drawn to that image of yourself, and the behaviour that goes with it. This is the 'towards' motivation that draws us to happiness and pleasure, and is the basis of the swish and similar

techniques. It accounts for the universal truism 'You are what you think about most'.

3. You get pleasant surprises as you go, such as finding that you smoke less without trying, you have more energy, confidence and control over your life.

Seen in this light, the motivation to quit is within your control. You can carry out the various visualisation exercises under your own steam, and create the inner experiences, or 'strategies', that motivate you. The more vivid and realistic you make your imagery, and the more you practise it, the more you will perfect your mental programmes – including your motivation strategy. Combined, these factors will increase your motivation to the point that you can hardly wait to carry out your decision.

Other specific methods can affect your motivation. For example, the meta- yes-ing and no-ing in the previous chapter is a very effective motivation strategy as well as a technique for behavioural change. Your 'yes strategy' is, in fact, a personal motivation strategy you have used successfully in the past and which you can now use as a resource to apply to stopping smoking. Your 'no strategy' works in the 'away from' direction, but provides the same resulting motivation. When a smoker is shocked into a decision to quit through the illness or death of a smoker friend, this is the very sort of mental strategy they unknowingly use. They make comments such as 'There is *no* way I am going to go that route'. They decide *no* to that eventuality in their own life. In the same way, a pregnant

woman says a resolute 'no' to any harm to her baby.
Likewise, by visualising yourself in three non-smoker
situations that support the new belief you chose (see Chapter
6), you create pleasurable mind pictures that draw you
towards their realisation, just like a dream holiday.

THE CHAIN OF FUNDAMENTALS

If you have read the book carefully so far, and carried out
the suggestions, you will be informed, prepared and
motivated for the final stage of making the break. In this
chapter we concentrate on the point of cessation, revising a
few major issues and offering tips about ensuring that you
stay free of cigarettes for life. First, a potted reminder of the
fundamentals of what you have learnt:

1. You need to be clear that you want to give up and why.
   Knowing that smoking is bad for you is not an adequate
   reason. Even knowledgeable medical people remain
   stuck in their habit. You need not wait for a Damascus
   road revelation – the book is designed to create the
   necessary focus.

2. You need to identify old beliefs that caused you to start
   smoking and kept you going until you became hooked.
   You can do this by simple recall, in a relaxed but
   focused, hypnotic mode. It's a memory exercise, but
   more intensive and purposeful than ordinary
   remembering.

3. You need to identify the reasons you continue to smoke
   today, such as the 'popular pretexts' we covered in detail
   in Chapter 4. The parts reconciliation exercise in

Chapter 6 and the self-understanding questions in Chapter 5 should have identified these, and also some forgotten factors under 2 above.

4. You then choose new beliefs to replace these outdated ones, and consider real reasons to change. These will form your new mental strategies and non-smoker identity.

5. You need to come to the point when you are not 'giving up' anything of value, or making any sacrifice. You will usually reach this point at some stage in the process as you stay open-minded. Otherwise, simply treat any niggling doubt as a belief change, reversing it to make it positive and useful. For example, in place of 'it helps me relax', state 'I am more and more relaxed as a healthy non-smoker'. Then visualise three behaviour scenarios that illustrate your new belief as we described in Chapter 6.

6. Change any unwanted mental programmes or strategies by doing the exercises in Chapter 6: belief change; reconciling conflicting 'parts'; and 'meta-yes-ing and no-ing'.

7. Prepare for stimulus-response type behaviour by identifying the sort of behaviour and situations that might cause you to relapse, and apply the swish exercise to 'anchor' a new, automatic association. You can test this out so that you are sure it works and you can rely on it in the most extreme temptation (see Chapter 6).

8. Make common-sense preparation to minimise the chances of being with people or in places where you are likely to face undue temptation in the days and weeks

after making your break. Plan your final break thoroughly – like a house move or a wedding. You don't want any crises or nasty surprises. We will remind you of some ideas below.

Treat these fundamentals as a chain of changes that will guarantee lifelong cessation from smoking. That means, of course, that the weakest link is critical, and may spell success or failure. But if you feel unsure about one or more of these major components of giving up, don't worry. Simply revisit the relevant sections in the book, do the exercises again and settle your mind one issue at a time. Or, for the sake of a few days, slowly re-read the book – it is worth getting it right for such big rewards. There is much to gain from not much effort, and the more you are prepared, the less effort you eventually need to expend relative to a successful, lifetime outcome. This is the smart method of understanding and using existing body-mind systems rather than doing it 'your way'.

In Chapter 1 we recommended keeping a smoking diary, and if you did this you should have some useful personal intelligence you can draw upon when planning the few weeks after you quit. For example, you may now know the precise people, places and circumstances that might precipitate a relapse, so you can make special plans to avoid them. At the very least, to be forewarned is to be forearmed, and a red light will flash as you meet these situations, giving you that invaluable few moments to take a few deep breaths and act rationally.

PLANNING FOR PERMANENT SUCCESS

Here are some ideas for your smoke-free plans. Some will have been taken account of in the non-smoking mental programmes you have created, while other suggestions may be new. It is not exhaustive anyway, and you may think of common-sense ideas that apply in your particular circumstances. In some cases you may wish to repeat the change exercises to incorporate issues you had not considered, and which will make your reprogramming more realistic.

Red lights

Identify difficult or tempting 'trigger' situations. Learn from past attempts to quit. What helped? What caused your relapse? Ask:

- What provokes me into having a cigarette
  - having a cup of coffee?
  - answering the telephone?
  - making a telephone call?
  - switching on the computer?
  - going to the pub?

- Who provokes me into smoking?

- On what sort of occasion?

- What are my most vulnerable times and days?

- As you think back, which cigarettes could you easily have not smoked? And why?

All this is invaluable intelligence. Register it as **red lights** in your mind. Writing this down will help.

Diary

Continue your smoker's diary if you have kept one. Record your triumphs and alleviate the black cloud times by freely expressing your private thoughts. Peruse your diary to identify 'red lights', and use it as a checklist for planning, and also to revive your motivation and commitment where necessary.

Places

You don't need to live your life avoiding places, but nor does it make sense to tempt fortune. After all, as a non-smoker the places you frequent will change naturally. So you can plan out of your life places you connect with smoking. Mentally check through places at work and away from work; places you frequent regularly, and those you go to just occasionally – especially places you might go to in the weeks immediately after giving up. Choose places that don't allow smoking. For example, Linda enjoyed going to the cinema (which was all non-smoking) and planned successive, marathon viewings to take her safely through many of the critical hours. She didn't smoke, of course, and thoroughly enjoyed herself into the bargain. Otherwise, go to a place you know has a non-smoking area and practise being a non-smoker. Plan to go to nice places and incorporate special treats.

People

Consider people who you usually smoke with at work,

socially and in your extended family. Decide on a specific strategy for each of these, including complete avoidance. Tell family, friends and colleagues you are about to stop and need their support. Especially solicit the help of your partner, and close friends whom you can rely on to act in your interests and support you all the way. If any are unhelpful or cynical, give them a wide berth for a while.

Eating and drinking

Identify any eating or drinking situation when you would normally smoke, whether daily at work, on special occasions, in the local pub, after work and so on. Bear in mind that alcohol will not help much during the critical withdrawal period, so it is well to avoid it for a while and plan your life accordingly. Better, for instance, to have a drink with non-smokers if you do drink in moderation. Drink plenty of fluid such as water or fruit juice. Change what you eat – for instance what you have for breakfast. Start a quality diet that involves new, exciting foods that will maintain your weight and health while giving a new interest. Suck sugar-free fruit gums or lollipops if you like them. Keep a supply with you and stick one in when you get the faintest hint of temptation. If you link smoking with drinking coffee, it makes sense to give up coffee first, as part of your planning.

Recurring events

These can be critical. For example, weekly or monthly work meetings, sports events, holidays such as Christmas and bank holidays when you might wind down and celebrate, and family visits. Identify these and decide on a strategy to either avoid them or have the necessary control of events to avoid needless temptation.

Travel

Consider travelling, such as by train, when you might normally light up. If you have to travel by train, choose the non-smoking carriage of course, rather than tempt fortune. Charles, after some 30 years as a heavy smoker, timed his break to coincide with a 25-hour flight to Australia over the millennium period, so was almost detoxified by the time he landed and got through the most important period without a whimper.

Rewards

Plan for rewards – they are great motivators. Reward yourself for every day you are free. Don't be stingy. Have a bigger reward after a week, a month and so on. Share it with someone you love. Think about what you can buy with the money you will save. Pamper yourself. Have a hair do, for instance, or arrange in advance to have your teeth checked and cleaned – prepare to look and feel good. Remind yourself often why you are quitting (have a card with a list of the pluses). Mental rewards can be as effective as material ones once you master visualisation techniques. Plan something enjoyable to do every day.

Routines

Change your routines. New mental programmes will help to confuse the old ones. In a new situation, such as a new job, you *expect* to act differently and are more ready for changes. For example, take a different route to work, change your lunch arrangements, go to bed early (sleep is ideal for stress-free detoxification and general wellbeing), drink tea instead of coffee or vice versa. This changes your focus and makes you *aware* of your behaviour, so that you don't succumb to old habits. Doing new things keeps your mind occupied. All this makes smoking-related habits just a part of the overall change, and keeps them in perspective.

Keep active

Keeping active also keeps your mind as well as body occupied. Clean the car. Do some housework. Change your activities frequently so that you never go on to 'autopilot' and act without thinking. One veteran smoker, Rod, coincided his final break with a big garden landscaping job over the weekend at the house of a non-smoking friend. He finished shattered, but exhilarated at managing without a cigarette. Do things specifically that you know reduce stress, such as taking a hot bath, listening to your favourite music, reading, enjoying a sport or jogging. Vary these a lot, so that you never have long enough to get bored and fidgety.

Problems

Take your mind off a problem and come back to it later. Take deep breaths frequently. This helps you relax and pumps lovely oxygen into your lungs and your brain. Avoid stressful situations. If your job is a main cause of stress, consider a few days' holiday. Once you get through the withdrawal period you will have more energy, a better perspective on problems and higher self-esteem.

Sleep

Try to go to bed earlier and get plenty of sleep. That's another eight or so hours of successful abstinence without even thinking about it. A lot of the repair work to your body happens when you are asleep. Just before dropping off to sleep is an ideal time to 'install' motivating non-smoker benefits.

Hands

Get things to hold in your hands – a good time for a new pen or watch to play with. Chew a pencil, file your nails (or bite them – it beats smoking), have a supply of little lollipops.

Cigarettes

Keep cigarettes away from you, including other people's. Be as ingenious as you might have been when planning not to be caught without cigarettes after the shops have closed. The same applies to ash trays, lighters and all the paraphernalia of smoking – out of sight, out of mind. Brute willpower doesn't work – adopt an avoidance strategy. Be smart and use your brain.

Date

Decide on a date and time to stop that will maximise your chances of success in view of all the above. Time it to a holiday, perhaps, or a special day such as a birthday or anniversary. Don't assume you have greater power of resistance than the millions who repeatedly fail. Some successful quitters plan their date to coincide with a long weekend, and others time their final break with a holiday, or even a scheduled period in hospital so that they (or others) have more control over their lives while withdrawing.

WHAT IF YOU HAVE A CIGARETTE?

Finally, what if, with all your preparation, you cave in and have a cigarette? Will it be all over again? No, but if you don't nip it in the bud, it may be. Hence the motto 'Not even a puff' – and that applies literally. Multiple tryers and failers all say that it was a single cigarette that ruined all their effort. As it happens, even if you failed to reprogramme all your smoking-related habits, you will have made enough changes to your brain circuitry to ensure that all kinds of warning lights and emotions will crowd your mind the instant you find yourself acting like a slave again. That momentary awareness is your chance. Stop mid-puff. It will take just a few seconds to take a few deep breaths, and while doing so remind yourself of the benefits of being a non smoker, triple images of the new 'you' and the motivating swish images.

Get away on your own as soon as you can, and re-do some of your belief change programmes. Say or mentally rehearse your new beliefs and reaffirm your yes and nos. Incorporate the specific circumstances (stimulus image) that triggered your relapse as a new swish pattern (see Chapter 6) to be confident you have plugged that gap. Check out your list of 'making the break' tips above. You will find your determination returns quickly to where it was – and even increases. You may feel exhilarated at having succeeded in a critical, testing moment. Almost certainly, having got through such a test, you have cracked your smoking dependency once and for all. If – or when – you are tempted you know the routine and you know that it works.

This last advice doesn't mean you should expect a relapse. On the contrary, that's why you have waited and prepared so thoroughly before finally making the break. But it does mean that even this eventuality is catered for, and even niggling doubts are taken care of. However, it is impossible to overestimate the importance of not succumbing to even a puff when freedom and so much more is within your reach ('a puff is enuff'!).

CESSATION SELF-SCRIPT

So that you can focus on the specific time you have set to start your non-smoking life, it will help to use a simple script designed to register the final break in your unconscious mind. In doing this, it will help if you remind yourself of the exercises you have already carried out in the same, trance-like state:

- identifying and changing the old beliefs
- reconciling the parts
- your yes and no commitments
- the motivating images of behaving in accordance with your new beliefs
- and the rapid swishes.

Remind yourself of these before you embark on the final script below. You should have done all the mental reprogramming in the exercises throughout the book anyway, so this final exercise just sets the starting clock.

If you can get someone to slowly read it out, so much the better. Or you can obtain a specially prepared cassette tape from the website at the end of this chapter. In either case you can close your eyes and become very open to the powerful suggestions to your subconscious mind. But with a little preparation you can make it a DIY job – such as by recording it and including excerpts from the exercises earlier if you need to remind yourself. Read it through first, before you decide on a method that suits you. Be sure to choose a place and time when you will not be interrupted and you can focus completely on the business in hand. Some people need the support of other people more than others. Most research shows that the chances of long-term success increase in line with the number of 'consultations' or the time spent with others getting help and support. This is where family and friends can help. Or you may want to arrange a consultation with one of the authors, or someone we can recommend near where you live. Check out the website and contact details on page 146.

You now have all the information you need to give up smoking once and for all. You will now understand yourself better, especially the way your unconscious mind has been at work in maintaining the smoking behaviour. You know how to clearly visualise yourself to create the new, non-smoking person. In the previous chapter you learnt how to change the programmes that run your different smoking-related habits. You have made a conscious decision to stop, so now you can make the final break.

Get into a relaxed state of mind, using the ten to one method in Chapter 5 or the method that works best for you. Go deeper – breathe slowly and deeply – feel yourself sinking – or maybe floating – think back to when you started smoking, and the reasons you started (state these, as identified earlier in Chapter 6) – but your life has changed in so many ways and now you want to be free from the power of cigarettes, to be healthy and confident – a non-smoker from this moment on – you have realised all the harm that smoking brings (state the top few you identified earlier) – now see yourself as a non-smoker – you look so healthy and confident, you feel free as you look around – seeing things through your own eyes – and notice how things are better – no more guilt – you have more choices – you hear yourself saying yes – *yes* – to your new non-smoker life – imagine those situations in which you would have reached for a cigarette and see yourself acting instead as the new, strong, confident, non-smoking person you have now become (go through a few swishes at this point: it takes literally a few seconds) – you wonder what there ever was to give up, as you have only gained – repeat some yes and no affirmations that come to mind and experience the confidence of success – get ready to come back to the present and enjoy the continuing feeling of being in control, free of cigarettes for ever – confident that in mind and body you are a changed person – completely free to be who you want to be and behave as you wish to – having said 'no' to smoking and all the habits connected with it, once and for all, and 'yes' to a cleaner, happier, healthier, future. From your whole mind and body say 'yes' to freedom – at the count of five you will be wide awake, feeling wonderful 1 – 2 – 3 coming right out – 4 – 5.

Congratulate yourself. Enjoy your achievement. Tell us about it. Look at yourself in the mirror and savour the pleasure of taking control of your life and creating a better future.

Keep this book handy, as well as your diary, so that you have plenty of helpful tips immediately available whenever you need them. Repeat your positive visualisation exercises and a few swishes whenever you wish to, as these will reinforce the change that has already taken place. Remember that it gets easier *every minute* that you go without a cigarette. Look forward to the rewards you have agreed to give yourself, and all the other benefits you have imagined as you have prepared for a better way of life.

CONTACT THE AUTHORS

Please let us know how you get on. Your story may help
many others. For further help, consultations on smoking
cessation, audio cd discs and details of No Smoking
Corporate Programmes, telephone:

Dr Karl Morris   Office: 00 +44 (0) 1925 764053
                           Mobile: 00 +44 (0) 7889 249031
Email   drkarlmorris@golf-brain.com
Website   www.golf-brain.com
Address   95 Common Lane, Culcheth,
                           Cheshire WA3 3HF

Index